DISEASES OF MAJOR MEDICINAL PLANTS

K.K. Jnardhanan

2018
Daya Publishing House®
A Division of
Astral International Pvt. Ltd.
New Delhi - 110 002

First Published, 2002
Reprinted, 2018

ISBN: 978-81-7035-264-8 (Hardbound)

Published by : **Daya Publishing House®**
A Division of
Astral International Pvt. Ltd.
– ISO 9001:2015 Certified Company –
4736/23, Ansari Road, Darya Ganj
New Delhi-110 002
Ph. 011-43549197, 23278134
E-mail: info@astralint.com
Website: www.astralint.com

Dedicated to the memory of my father
Kainoor Krishnankutty

ACKNOWLEDGEMENTS

I wish to express my sincere thanks to Dr. P. Pushpangadan, Director, Tropical Botanic Garden and Research Institute, Thiruvananthapuram (presently Director, National Botanical Research Institute, Lucknow) for providing me all facilities for undertaking this work and also for his help and encouragement during the preparation of this monograph.

I gratefully acknowledge the generous financial support of Department of Science and Technology, New Delhi, Government of India, under their USERS Scheme for undertaking this work and but for this support it would have not been possible to bring out this monograph.

I am grateful to Dr. V. George, Deputy Director, TBGRI, Thiruvananthapuram for his unqualified help and co-operation during this work.

During the preparation of this book, I have been permitted the generous use of the library and CD-ROM facilities of M.S. Swaminathan Research Foundation, Chennai, Kerala Forest Research Institute (KFRI), Peechi, Thrissur and Kerala Agricultural University, Vellanikara, Thrissur and Centre for Advance Studies in Botany, University of Madras, Chennai. Facilites provided by these institutes are gratefully acknowledged.

I also thank Dr. K.V. Sankaran, Scientist, KFRI, Peechi and Dr. S. Rajasekharan, Deputy Director, Shri K.M.A. Rahman, Registrar and Shri Ravi Abraham, Administrative Officer, TBGRI, Thiruvananthapuram for their help and co-operation during course of this work.

My sincere thanks are also due to Shri Baby Yohannan, Central Institute of Medicinal and Aromatic Plants, Lucknow for typing the final version of the manuscript and to Miss N. Sheena for technical help and Shri Anil Mittal, M/s. Daya Publishing House, Delhi for publishing this work.

K.K. Janardhanan
Tropical Botanic Garden and
Research Institute
Thiruvananthapuram

FOREWORD

In spite of the tremendous progress in the development of modern medicine, plants continue to be an important source of drugs throughout the world, particularly in the developing countries. The last two decades registered significant revival in the use of higher plants for health care and treatment of several diseases for which modern medicine was not found effective. Because of this, demand for plant drugs enhanced enormously. This has necessitated in the large-scale cultivation of a number of medicinal plants in the recent years in order to maintain sustainable supply to the pharmaceutical industries. Extensive cultivation of these plants has increased the pathological problems. The diseases of these plants and their intensity have increased to a great extent.

A number of books on the chemistry, pharmacognosy and utilization of medicinal plants have been brought out during the last two decades. However, no comprehensive publication on the diseases of these plants and their management has been published. Therefore, this monograph on the disease of major medicinal plants is a timely contribution. Dr. K.K. Janardhanan, former Deputy Director and Head, Microbiology and Plant Pathology Division, Central Institute of Medicinal and Aromatic Plants, Lucknow has several years of experience on the disease of medicinal plants to his credit. He is an acknowledged expert in this field. I earnestly hope that this monograph will be of significant use to students, teachers and researchers in this area as well as to growers of medicinal plants. I congratulate Dr. Janardhanan for bringing out this useful publication.

Akhtar Husain, FNA, FNASc
Former Director
Central Institute of Medicinal and
Aromatic Plants
Lucknow

PREFACE

The importance of plants as a major source of therapeutic agents has assumed greater importance during the recent years because of the remarkable revival in use of plants for health care in the last two decades throughout the world. This has resulted in the large-scale exploitation of some medicinal plants as raw materials for pharmaceuticals. In order to obtain sustainable supply large scale cultivation of a large number of medicinal plants was necessitated. As a result, commercial cultivation of a large number of medicinal plants has been taken up in recent years in several countries.

Specialized commercial cultivation of medicinal plants has increased their pathological problems. The diseases of these plants and their intensity have multiplied. A number of books on the chemistry, pharmacognosy, agrotechnology and utilization of medicinal plants have been published in the recent years. However, no book of the diseases of medicinal plants is available. Hence, there is a pressing need for comprehensive publication on this subject. The information presented in this book represents knowledge accumulated by me over a period of several years of experience in this area. I am particularly indebted to Dr. Akhtar Husain, Former Director, Central Institute of Medicinal and Aromatic Plants, Lucknow in whose laboratory and guidance I gained much of this experience.

I have attempted to present the available information on diseases of important medicinal plants caused by fungi, bacteria, viruses and nematodes in this book. Physiological disturbances caused by non-parasitic factors are often as destructive as those caused by well-recognized parasitic organisms. No attempt has been made to provide information on this aspect and also on those damages caused by insects in this book. A number of important medicinal plants do not find place in the list of plants included in this book, because no serious disease has been reported on them. However, it is my earnest hope that the information contained in this book will be valuable to students, teachers and research workers in this field and the application of the knowledge will benefit the growers.

K.K. Janardhanan
Tropical Botanic Gardens and
Research Institute
Thiruvananthapuram

CONTENTS

INTRODUCTION

Medicinal plants have been used as a major source of therapeutic agents by human beings for thousands of years. Ancient man obtained more than 90% of his medicaments from higher plants. However, the importance of plants as a source of drugs decreased to certain extent with the advancement of knowledge in modern medicine and especially because of the phenomenal development in synthetic drugs and antibiotics. A large number of active constituents of plants were synthesised and it was more or less assumed that most of the plant drugs would be sooner or later obtained from synthetic sources. Inspite of the fact that synthetic drugs and antibiotics brought out a revolution in controlling different diseases of man and animals, plants continued to occupy an important place as raw material for some most important drugs used in modern medicine throughout the world (Husain, 1993).

According to Farnsworth even in a highly developed country like United States of America, more than 25 per cent of the prescription were found to contain one or more plant products. More than 100 active constituents obtained from different species of plants were found to be used in these prescriptions (Husain, 1993). During the last twenty years, there has been a complete transformation of medicinal system in the world and specially in those countries of the West which were totally dependent on modern medicine. Because of the realistion of toxicity associated with the use of antibiotics and synthetic drugs, the western society is obsessed with the idea that drugs from natural sources are safer, as compared to synthetics. The importance of plants as a major source of clinical agents is much more in developing countries of Asia, Africa and South America, where traditional medicine is practised widely. There has been considerable revival in the use of higher plants for health care purposes during the last 2 decades throughout the world. Considerable emphasis has also been laid in the research programme of drug companies during the last 10 years to tap the plant kingdom for treatment of such diseases for which the modern medicine does not have any effective treatment. These include virus diseases like herpes, AIDS, cancer, arthritic disorders, liver ailments, among others (Handa, 1992, Bhakuni and Jain, 1995). The entire world and especially the developed world has been swept by a green wave where common man has a feeling that anything from nature is safer as compared to those obtained from synthetic sources. More and more people are switching over to plant drugs, herbal health foods and herbal teas in Europe and the United States for treatment of common ailments. More than 100 plants are used in modern medicine and the number of plants used in indigenous systems of medicine is well over 200.

Steroidal drugs are one of the most important groups of chemicals having wide use all over the world. Although steroids are used for treatment of more than 90 different human disorders, their most common use is in the form of sex hormones, corticosteroids, oral contraceptive and anabolic agents. These drugs can be obtained either by total synthesis or by partial synthesis from animals and plant products. Various raw materials, which are used for production of these steroids, are cholesterol and bile acids from animals, stigmasterol and Beta-sitosterol from soyabean oil and other plants as well as steroidal sapogenins from plants. Various plant sapogenins used as raw material in medicine today are diosgenin, hecogenin and solasodine. The most important raw material for the synthesis of steroidal drugs is diosgenin which is obtained from species of *Dioscorea*.

A number of opium alkaloids such as morphine, codeine, papaverine and nascopine are extensively used in medicine. Except papaverine, which is also obtained from synthetic sources, all other alkaloids are still obtained from opium poppy (*Papaver somniferum*) either from latex or from direct extraction of the poppy husk or straw.

The bark of the *Cinchona* tree contains 6-7% total alkaloids. Although a large number of alkaloids are found in *Cinchona*, the most important are quinine and quinidine. While quinine is used as an antimalarial, quinidine is employed as a cardiac depressant to control auricular fibrillation (antiarrhythmic agent). At one time the use of quinine as antimalarial had gone down and the production of this alkaloid also decreased considerably. However, because of the development of the resistant strains of malarial parasite to synthetic antimalarials, use of quinine has increased recently and it is expected that in the countries of Asia and Africa, specially because of recurrence of malaria, particularly caused by resistant strains of the malarial parasite, use of quinine has considerably increased in the third world. Similarly, quinidine employed as antiarrhythmic agent, also has increased demand with the development of better health care facilities in the third world.

The crude drug senna is obtained from the leaves and pods of *Cassia angustifolia*, often referred as Indian Senna, and *C. acutifolia* designated as Alexandrian Senna. Sennosides are important laxative used in medicine.

Psyllium husk is obtained from ripe seeds of *Plantago ovata*. The seed husk is used in medicine because of its mucilage, which is colloidal in nature and serves as a safe bulk-laxative.

Tropane alkaloids, which include hyoscyamine, hyoscine and atropine, are some of the most commonly used phytochemicals in modern medicine mainly because of their anticholinergic, antispasmodic and pain relieving properties. These are commonly used for treatment of a number of diseases affecting respiratory and intestinal tract. Various plants which are used as source of these alkaloids are *Datura* species, *Hyosycamus* species, *Atropa* species and *Duboisia* species.

Various species of *Rauvolfia* have been used as source of hypotensive alkaloids. The most common species being exploited, are *Rauvolfia serpentina* and *R. vomitoria*. Although roots of *Ravolfia* contain more than three dozen alkaloids, the most important alkaloids are reserpine, rescinnamine and deserpidine from *R. serpentina* and reserpine and ajmaline from *R. vomitoria*. The hypotensive alkaloids from *R. serpentina* and *R. vomitoria* are used for treatment of high blood-pressure as well as tranquillizers. The demand for pure alkaloids of *Rauvolfia* has gone down recently. However, demand for total extract and the root powder is still fairly high.

Although there are a number of plants, which contain cardiac glycosides, the two most important plants containing these glycosides, are *Digitalis purpurea* and *D. lanata*. *Digitalis purpurea* is used only to a limited extent and most of the present supply of cardiac glycosides is obtained from the leaves of *D. lanata* which contain digoxin and lanatoside-C.

Liquorice consists of dried roots and rhizomes of *Glycyrrhiza glabra*. The main active constituents of the drug are saponin like glycosides of which glycyrrhizin is most important. In the form of crude extract, it is used as ...ctorant and anti-inflammatory as well as demulscent to improve the flavour of various bitter medicinal preparations. Purified extract and carbexonolone is also used for treatment of gastric and duodenal ulcers. Pure glycyrrhetic acid is also used for treatment of skin diseases as well as peptic ulcers.

Common periwinkle (*Catharanthus roseus*) is one plant, which has become important in modern medicine during the last 15-20 years. The drug is obtained both from the leaves as well as roots of the plant. The plant contains more than 100 alkaloids, ajmalicine (raubasine), an alkaloid obtained from the roots is of considerable use in modern medicine. The alkaloid has been used as a vasodialator for controlling auricular fibrillation. Leaves of the plant contain two anticancer alkaloids; viz. vincristine and vinblastine which are drug of choice for the treatment of several types of cancers.

Podophyllum resin obtained from *Podophyllum* species are lignan glycosides called podophyllotoxin. Two derivatives of podophyllotoxin, called etoposide and teniposide have been recommended for the treatment of various types of cancers.

A new hypotensive drug, forskolin was developed from *Coleus forskohlii*. Pharmacological studies of *C. forskohlii* led to the isolation of deterpenoid, forskolin. The drug is claimed to be one of the most effective drugs for the treatment of cardiovascular diseases.

Plants suffer from diseases cause of which are similar to those affecting animals and man. Plant growth and yield depend on protecting the plants from diseases. Anything that affects the health of plants is likely to affect their growth and yield and also seriously reduce their usefulness to mankind. Plant diseases are thus important to man because they not only damage plants but also the plant products. Plant diseases are caused by fungi, bacteria, mycoplasmas, viruses, viroids, nematodes, protozoa and parasitic higher plants apart from environmental and physiological factors.

There are several kinds of diseases affecting the plants and each crop plant can be affected by a number of diseases. Disease condition in the plants are recognized according to the symptoms produced by the pathogens. The usual disease symptoms are root rots, cankers, wilts, leaf spots, scabes, blights, anthracnoses, rusts, mildews, smuts, mosaic, yellows, root-knots, etc. Diseases caused by bacteria, fungi, nematodes, viruses and mycoplasma are characterized by the presence of these pathogens on the tissues of these plants. The presence of such pathogens at an active site on the surface of the plant would indicate that they are probably the cause of the disease. The presence of parasitic nematodes, fungal mycelium and spores or bacteria on the affected area of the diseased plants must be considered the possibilities of their role in the disease causation. The diagnosis of diseases caused by viruses, mycoplasma-like organisms is much more difficult and complicated. However, diagnosis of such diseases is primarly based on symptoms and transmission of the pathogen from diseased to healthy plants. Diseases of plants, thus, can be identified by the symptoms and the presence of the pathogen especially on the site of infection.

Causal Agents of Plant Diseases

Bacteria : Several plant diseases have been reported to be caused by bacteria. Numerous and excellent contributions on bacterial diseases of plants established the importance of bacteria as plant pathogens. Bacteria are minute, relatively simple, single celled organisms whose genetic material is not enclosed in a nuclear membrane. For this reason they are called procaryotes. Bacterial cells generally appear in one or several shapes. Bacillus (rod shaped) coccus (spherical or ovoid) and spiral (corkscrew or curved) are most common shapes. Individual bacteria may from pairs, chains or other groupings. Such formations are usually characteristic of particular species. Bacteria are enclosed in cell wall that are largely composed of substance called peptidoglycans. Bacteria generally reproduce by dividing into two equal daughter cells, the process is called binary fission. Many bacteria can move by using appendages called flagella. For nutrition, most bacteria use organic chemicals, which in nature can be derived from other dead organisms or from living hosts.

Fungi : Fungi are eucaryotes, the cells have distinct nucleus that contain genetic material and is surrounded by a special envelope called nuclear membrane. Fungi are unicellular or multicellular. True fungi have cell walls composed primarily of a substance called chitin. The unicellular forms of fungi are larger than bacteria. The most typical fungi are molds which form long filamentous and branched mycelia. Fungi can reproduce sexually or asexually. They obtain nourishment from their environment such as soil, water, animal or plant hosts. Classification of fungi is based largely upon the type of spores or fruiting body produced by them. The fungi are classified into four main classes: Zygomycota, Ascomycota, Basidiomycota and Deuteromycota. Zygomycota are characterized by the absence of cross walls in the multinucleate vegetative hyphae. In most cases sexual spore is formed. The downy mildews are example of this group. Ascomycota have septate hyphae and produce their sexual spores in a sac-like structure, the ascus. These spores are called ascospores. The asexual spores, conidia are usually produced during the parasitic phase on the host plant. Basidiomycota are characterized by the production of a basidium on which ordinarily four basidiospores are produced. The rusts, smuts and mushrooms belong to this group. Deuteromycota (fungi imperfecti) is a name applied to a group of fungi which for the most part are similar to ascomycota, except that they neither produce ascospores nor this stage has not been discovered.

Viruses : Viruses are so small that most can be seen only with an electron microscope and they are not cellular. They are structurally very simple : a virus particle contains a core made of only one type of nucleic acid, either DNA (deoxyribonucleic acid) or RNA (ribonucleic acid). This core is surrounded by a protein coat. Sometimes the coat is encased by an additional layer, a lipid membrane called an envelope. Viruses can reproduce only inside the cells of other organisms. Thus, all viruses are obligate parasites.

Studies on plant viruses had the beginning in 1886 when Mayer reproduced the tobacco mosaic disease by injecting the juice from infected tobacco plants into healthy plants. Beijerink in 1898 concluded that tobacco mosaic was caused by an unknown entity which he called virus. In 1935, Stanley isolated the infectious crystalline virus and concluded that the virus could be considered as a nucleo-protein which could multiply within a living cell. Viruses are able to infect plants in which they can multiply and cause well defined diseases. They can be transmitted from plant to plant. Unlike most bacteria and fungi, viruses cannot be cultivated in the laboratory and they multiply only in the living cells of the host plants.

Nematodes : Nematodes that attack plants are minute, slender microscopic worms. Because of their shape and the way they move, they are sometimes called eelworms. The first parasitic nematode was reported by Needham in 1743 within wheat galls. Studies by Cobb in 1913 to 1932 contributed greatly to the taxonomy, morphology and pathology of plant parasitic nematodes. The nematodes that cause disease in plants are obligate parasites, requiring living plants to obtain their food in order to grow and reproduce. A few of them can be reared in the laboratory in culture of fungi and on those parts where they can establish their usual parasitic relationship. Nematodes may be endoparasites, feeding chiefly inside the plant or ectoparasites feeding on the plant surface. Despite their small size, these nematodes are complex animals that have well-defined internal organs with special functions. Nematodes reproduce by laying eggs.

The anatomy of nematodes is simpler than other animal forms. The body of the adult male is usually cylindrical, filiform and tapering at each end. At the anterior end is the mouth, provided with papillae, leading to buccal cavity which in turn leads to oesophagus. The entire body is covered with smooth or transversely striated cuticle within a cuticular and muscular layer. The cavity between the wall and body organs is filled with colourless liquid. Early in the development, the nematodes differentiate into male and female forms. The females are saccate, pyriform, pear shaped oval or round. After copulation the body becomes filled with eggs in a jelly-like sac. The eggs are elliptical and colourless. The eggs may be held in the body of females, which then become cyst or may be exuded out in a mass. Differentiation of the larvae takes place within the egg and second stage larvae hatch out to develop into adults after several moulting.

Mycoplasma : Doi and co-workers in 1967 observed mycoplasma like bodies in the phloem of plants infected with several leafhopper–transmitted diseases in Japan. They resemble bacteria in some respect. They lack cell walls. They are highly pleomorphic. In 1972 Davis and his colleagues observed the association of spiroplasma with corn stunt disease. Spiroplasma resembles mycoplasma and bacteria in some respects. Mycoplasma cells are very small, ranging in size from 0.1 to 0.25 μm.

Viroid : Diener in 1971, observed that potato spindle tuber disease was caused by a small molecule of infectious ribonucleic acid, which he called a viroid. Viroids are smallest known infectious agents. Several plant diseases are known to be caused by viroids.

General Symptoms of Diseases

Mildew : Mildews are diseases in which growth of the pathogen is seen on the surface of the host. The disease appeares as white, grey, brownish or puplish patches of varying sizes on leaves, stems or fruits. In downy mildew the superficial growth is cottony or downy layer, while in powdery mildew profuse superficial growth of the fungus with enormous number of spores are formed, giving a dusty powdery appearance.

Rust : The symptoms have rusty appearance. The rusts appear as relatively small pustules of spores, usually breaking through the host epidermis. The pustules may be red, brown, yellow or black in colour.

Necrosis : In this condition death of cells, tissues and organ occur. The dead areas show characteristic appearance in different hosts.

Spots : The cells are killed in a definite limited areas and dead tissue usually turn to different shades of brown. The shape of lesions on leaves or fruits may be round, angular or irregular. The dead areas are often surrounded by red, purple, yellow or brown margins.

Canker : A canker is a dead area in the bark or cortex of the stems especially of woody plants. Canker vary in size and often definitely margined. The surface may be smooth or rough and usually sunken. Superficial layers of the tissues are initially affected. The dead bark splits and finally peels off. The affected branches or the whole plant often die.

Blight : The symptoms refer to sudden death of plants or their leaves, blossoms or twigs. The dead organ usually turns brown or black leading to burnt appearance.

Damping-off : The stem is atttacked near the soil surface. The affected portions become weak and is unable to stand in an erect posture. This results in toppling down and death of seedlings.

Rot : The affected tissues decompose and turn brown. The cell walls are mostly disintegrated. Fleshy tissues of stems, roots, leaves, flowers, buds and fruits are affected. Depending upon dissolution brought about by the pathogen, the rots may be grouped as soft-rot, wet-rot or dry-rot. According to the organ attacked the rots may be called root-rot, stem-rot, bud-rot or fruit-rot.

Wilts : The leaves and other green or succulent parts lose their trugidity, become flaccid and droop. The effect is usually seen first in some leves and young growing tips. The whole plant may suddenly wilt and dry up. Wilting may of be the result of injury to root system or plugging of water conducting vessels.

Die-back : The symptoms are characterised by drying stems or branches from tip to the base.

Galls : These are malformations of irregular shapes more or less globose due to disorganized growth. Fleshy or woody tissues of stem and roots are affected.

Curl : The leaves twisted, curled and distorted due to growth in tissues in localised areas of the leaf.

Witches'-broom : Numerous slender branches arise from particular regions in clusters giving an appearance of broom. The leaves become narrow. The flowers are transformed to small leaves. These symptoms are often referred to little leaf or phyllody.

Any disturbance brought about by a pathogen or an environmental factor interfere with normal physiological functions of plants. Affected cells and tissues of diseased plants are usually weakened or destroyed by the pathogen. The kind of cells and tissue that are infected, determine the type of physiological functions of the plant that will be interferred. Thus, infection of roots interferes with absorption of water and translocation of nutrients. Infection of foliage interferes with photosynthesis, infection of cortex interferes with translocation of photosynthetic products and infection of flower and fruits interferes with reproduction. Affected cells and tissues of diseased plants are usually weakened or destroyed. The ability of such cells and tissues to perform their normal physiological functions especially the secondary metabolite biosynthesis is drastically reduced. Medicinal plants are affected by a large number of diseases caused by fungi, bacteria, nematodes, viruses and mycoplasma. These diseases are important because they significantly affect the physiological functions of the plants. Thus, the diseases directly are concerned with the manufacture of plant products, phytochemicals and pharmaceuticals.

1
BELLADONNA

Belladonna (*Atropa belladonna* L. and *Atropa acuminata* Royle ex Lendle) is a perennial herb. The drug belladonna is obtained from the flowering tops and roots. Belladonna was known to ancient people of Mesopotamia (1500-2000 B.C.) (Husain, 1993). *Atropa belladonna* occurs naturally in Central and Southern Europe. It is cultivated in a number of countries including England, Germany, Poland, Czechoslovakia, Hungary, Russia, USA and India. *Atropa acuminata* occurs naturally in North-western Himalayas in Jammu and Kashmir and Himachal Pradesh. Leaves and roots of belladonna contains alkaloids, such as 1-hyoscyamine, atropine and hyoscine. The plants find use in pharmaceutical industry as total belladonna alkaloids, extracts, tincture and plasters. Belladonna alkaloids are used in medicine because of their anticholinergic, antispasmodic and mydriatic properties. The natural drug and their derivatives are also used as sedative and tranquilizers. Belladonna is cultivated on commercial scale in several parts of the world. The crop is reported to be affected by a number of diseases caused by fungi and viruses.

1. Leaf Spots

Belladonna is reported to be affected by two leaf spot diseases, leaf necrosis (Ganguly and Pandotra, 1962) and leaf spot (Singh and Singh 1984). Leaf necrosis was reported from India and also from Argentina.

Symptoms : The symptoms consisted of greyish, white irregular spots with slight depression on the upper surface of the leaves. Later these spots coalesced and became necrotic resulting in defoliation and finally leading to the death of the plants. Pycnidia containing pycniospores have often been found on necrotic spots. The disease caused heavy loss to the yield and foliage production. The spots are mainly confined to the upper surface of the leaves. Severe infection resulted in drying and death of leaves.

Causal organism : *Ascochyta atropae* Bres. Pycnidia found on the spots are globose to oval, immersed in necrotic tissue, light brown, ostiolate, without a beak, 100.3 x 88.6 (86.1-115.6 x 68.9-110.7) µm. Spores cylindrical with rounded ends, rarely oval, straight, hyaline, pinkish in mass, 2-celled, rarely 3-celled, 8.9-3.1 (6.8-11.5x2.5-3.7) µm.

Control : Studies have shown that six sprays of Blitox-50 (Copper oxychloride) might be able to control the disease. The best control was reported by the application of Blitox-50 followed by Bavistin and Dithane Z-78 (Singh *et.al.*, 1985).

A leaf spot disease of belladonna was reported from U.S.A. (Fenne, 1954). The symptoms consisted of angular to round brown spots with chestnut coloured margins on the margins of the leaves. Generally the spots measured 1.5 to 4.5 µm. The disease was observed in India also (Singh and Singh, 1984).

Causal organisms : Cercospora atropae Kuashmina. The conidiophores are produced on the spots in tufts. They are olive brown in colour. Conidia are clavate, cylindrical, broadly rounded at the base and tapered towards the apex.

2. Roots-Rots

A number of fungi have been reported to cause root-rot diseases of belladonna. *Pythium* root-rot has been reported to be one of the serious diseases of this crop.. The disease is found epiphytotic in commercial plantations in Jammu and Kashmir. The disease appeared in the beginning of summer when day temperature started increasing beyond 30°C and the disease remained prevalent upto the end of September. Nearly 16-20% plants were observed to be affected. Both young nursery plants and older plants were affected.

Symptoms : The symptoms were sudden wilting of the aerial portions leading to drying and death of plants. The basal portion of the stem and roots showed browning and extensive disintegration of cortical tissues (Janardhanan *et.al.*, 1974).

Casual organisms : Pythium butleri Subramaniam. Grows rapidly on agar. Mycelium white, copious and robust, especially on the host; hyphae upto 9 μm diam; appresoria abundant, clustered with spherical ends; in the host inter and intra-cellular without haustoria. Zoosporangia, produced only in liquid culture, composed of lateral hyphal elements 40-150 μm long, with basal part crowded with upto 6 lobulate branches, the apical region tapering from 15 μm in width to 6 μm at the tip, where the contents pass into an apical vesicle before the zoospores are formed, encysted zoospores 11 μm diam, germinating by hyphae or by a single zoospore. Oogonia usually abundant in the host and produced readily in agar culture on shorter (4 μm) or longer (upto 70 μm) lateral hyphae; 15-33 μm diam wall colourless thin and smooth. Antheridia usually single, intercalary, commonly diclinous, rarely monoclinous, the hyphal part 9-22 μm long, the inflated part 10-17 μm deep, barrel-shapped or irregularly lobed, broadly applied to the oogonium, with little or no tapering, persistent. Oospores very loose in the oogonium 22.5 µm diam, wall smooth, colourless or slightly yellowish, and 2 µm thick; when mature has one central hyaline globule.

Pythium butleri causing root-rot of belladonna was reported to produce a heat stable toxic metabolite and pectolytic enzymes. The sudden wilting of infected plants and extensive disintegration during pathogenesis were due to the toxic metabolite and pectolytic enzymes produced by the pathogen (Janardhanan and Husain, 1974).

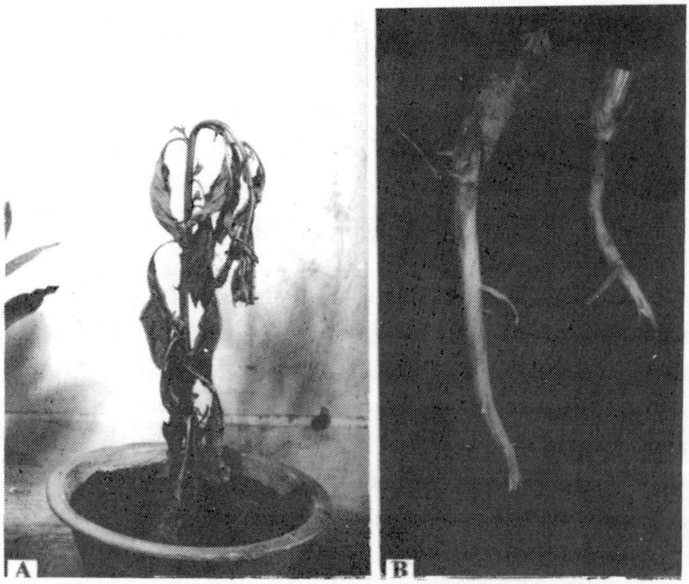

Fig. 1 : Root rot of *Belladonna* caused by *P. butleri* (A) infected plant (B) infected roots

Control : Drenching of seedlings in nursery with Dithane Z-78, Dexon or Benlate was found to control the disease. Fumigation of the soil with methyl bromide and treatment of seeds with Captan are also recommended for the control. Cultural practices such as avoiding excessive irrigation and crop rotation were useful to check the incidence of the disease.

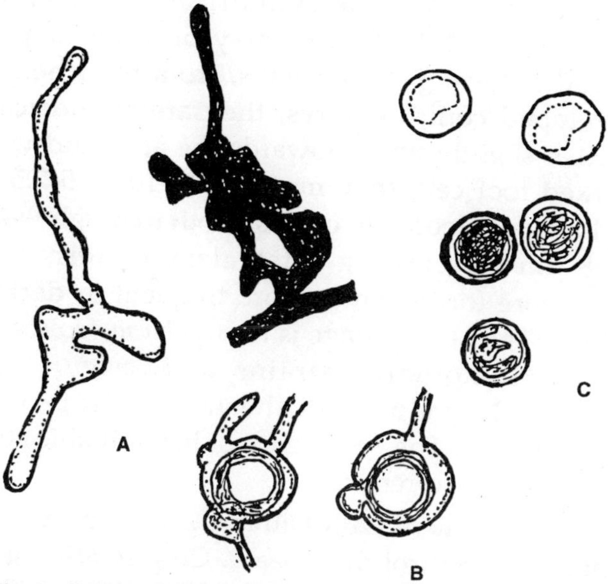

Fig. 2 : *P. butleri* - (A) sporangia (B) oogonia with antheridum (C) oogonium and oospores

Root-rot caused by *Fusarium* was observed as serious threat in the commercial plantations in Jammu and Kashmir. Nearly 40% of the plants were affected by the disease.

Symptoms : The symptoms consisted of yellowing of the leaves followed by wilting dehydration and death of plants. Root stem region of infected plants showed extensive disintegration of cortical tissue. Mature and full grown plants before or after flowering were more susceptible for infection (Janardhanan and Husain, 1974).

Casual organism : *Fusarium solani* (Mart) Sacc. Optimum temperature for growth and conidia formation in culture is 28°C. Growth on agar moderately rapid in 4-6 days with a somewhat sparse, floccose, greyish-white mycelium. Typically a bluish to bluish-brown discolouration develops in the agar. Microconidia form abundantly in the aerial mycelium from elongated lateral phialides; they are hyaline cylindrical wedge-shaped allantoid, 9-16 x 2-4 μm and may become septate. Macroconidia develop in 4-7 days, from branched and well developed conidiophores; they are cylindrical to falcate, often slightly wider towards the apex and with a well marked foot cell; they measure 40-100 x 5-7.5 μm. Chlamydosproes globose to oval, smooth to rough walled, 10-11 x 8 μm developing intercalary or terminally. Chlamydospore formation is more frequent in darkness than in light. The perfect stage is *Nectria haematococca* Berk & Broome. Homothallic strains of *F. solani* occur frequently and produce perithecia in culture under suitable conditions. The occurrence of heterothallic strains of this species is also reported.

Control : Treatment with Dithane Z-78 or Benlate has been reported to control the disease. Crop rotation is also recommended to be beneficial to check the disease (Sastry *et.al.*, 1977).

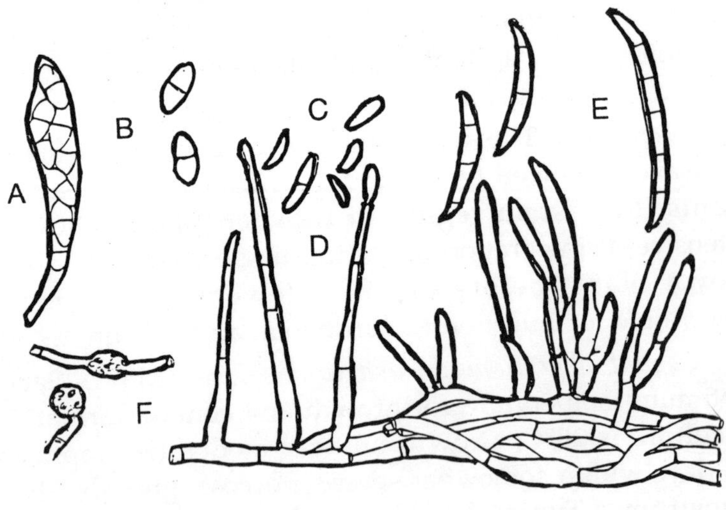

Fig. 3 : *F. solani* - (A) ascus (B) ascospores (C) microconidia (D) conidiophores (E) macroconidia (F) chlamydospores

Root-rot of belladonna caused by a number of species of *Phytophthora* has been reported. Thakur and Bhat (1974) reported a root-rot of belladonna in Kashmir valley caused by *Phytophthora nicotianae* Bide Haan *nicotianae*. The visible symptoms appeared first on the aerial parts.

Symptoms : Drooping of young leaves and branches, yellowing of older leaves and drying of whole apical portion of the plants or partial drying of leaves of some branches were typical symptoms of the diseases. The infection developed initially in the collar region and then on root and stem. The infected stems were yellowish brown in colour and root were dirty brown (Thakur and Bhat, 1974).

Phytophthora erythroseptica Pethybr. was reported to cause pink rot of belladonna in England. The disease was severe in Scotland during summer months. Alcock (1926) named the pathogen as *P. erythoseptica*. Middleton (1943) observed root and stem rot of *A. belladonna*. The disease was found to be caused by *P. parasitica* Dastur.

Control : Application of chloropicrin, Bordeaux mixture (2:2:50) or any offer copper fungicide were found effective to control the disease. Raising of the nursery on raised beds and avoidance of excess irrigation and crop rotation were found useful as preventive measures (Sastry *et.al.*, 1977). Seed treatment with Captan or Agrosan GN was also found to be effective to minimize the disease incidence (Husain and Janardhanan, 1967).

3. Collar Rot

The disease mainly affected the seedling. The infection normally starts at collar region as elongated water soaked lesions which girdle entire stem ultimately resulting in toppling of the plants. The decay of roots is followed by wilting and drooping of foliage. Severely infected plants invariably died (Sharma and Jandaik, 1979).

Causal organism : *Rhizoctonia solani* Kuhn.

4. Belladonna Mosaic

Smith (1943) described a new virus disease on *A. belladonna*. The virus is sap transmissible to tobacco and other solanaceous plants. The virus is inactivated at temperatures between 75-80°C. Sap extracted from infected plants remained active for 6-11 days.

Causal organism : Belladonna mosaic virus. Belladonna plants showing similar symptoms of belladonna mosaic virus has also been reported. Sol *et.al.*, (1961) showed that belladonna mosaic virus and rattle virus are transmitted by nematodes. Belladonna acts as a symptomless carrier of *Hyoscyamus* virus.

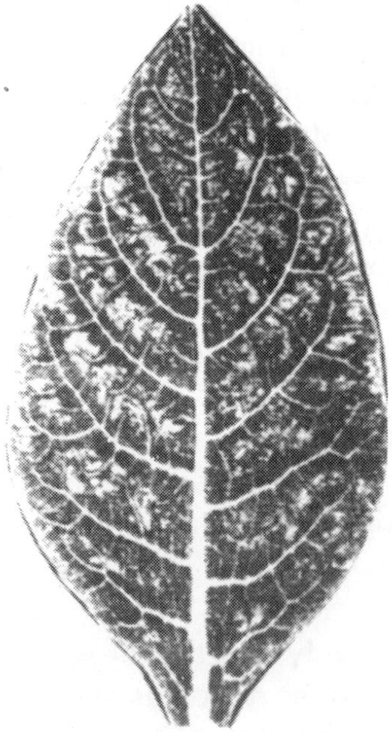

Fig. 4 : Symptoms of belladonna mottle virus infection

5. Belladonna Mottle

Belladonna mottle caused by a virus was first reported from Europe (Marcus, 1959). The virus was then reported in Germany on belladonna (Paul *et.al.*, 1968). The virus was also isolated from other plants in North America (Moline and Fries, 1972; Lee *et.al.*, 1979). Belladonna mottle virus was found in Czechoslovakia on spontaneously infected *A. belladonna*. The isolate is serologically distinct from the Hungarian isolate (Pelikanova *et.al.*, 1992).

The virus caused mild mottling and sometimes deformation in *A. belladonna*. The naturally infected plants were often found in the plant community. The infected plants showed severe mosaic, mottling and vein banding symptoms. The virus is readily transmitted by sap inoculation and by beetle and insect species. When tested by sap inoculation most of the solanaceous plants were infected systemically. Symptom expression in all hosts is variable.

Causal organism : Belladonna mottle virus (BML). Belladonna mottle virus is a RNA-containing virus with isometric particles approximately 2 nm which sediments as two components when centrifuged. The virus is strongly immunogenic. The serological relationship between the strains is very close. Physical data, RNA base composition and serological behaviour show that the virus belonged to the Andean potato latent virus subgroup of turnip yellow mosaic virus (Jankulowa, *et.al.*, 1968, Koenig, 1969). The virus is inactivated when heated at 80°C for 10 min. The virus retained its infectivity in the sap from infected plants for 5 days to 3 weeks. The virus is stable. The particles are isometric with angular polygonal outlines. The virus apparently has a structure similar to that of turnip yellow mosaic virus.

2
CINCHONA

Cinchona species are shrubs or trees upto 30 m tall. A dozen species of *Cinchona* are used in medicine as a source of cinchona alkaloids, namely quinine or quinidine. Only four or five species are commercially cultivated. They are *C. ledgeriana* Moens & Tremen, *C. officinalis* L, *C. calisaya* Wedd. and *C. succirubra* Pav. ex Kl. *Cinchona calisaya* is a large tree, *C. ledgeriana* and *C. officinalis* are slender trees and *C. succirubra* is a fast growing tree. All species of *Cinchona* are indigenous to tropical South American countries such as Bolivia, Peru, Costa Rica, Ecuador and Columbia and Asia and Africa. The plant was introduced to Indonesia by Dutch and to India by British Governments. The first plantation of *C. ledgeriana* was raised in Nilgiris of Tamil Nadu and later in Darjeeling district of West Bengal. *Cinchona* was also later introduced to Sri Lanka and to African countries (Husain, 1993). More than 30 quinoline alkaloids have been isolated from the bark of the stem, branches and roots of *Cinchona* species. Important alkaloids are quinine, quinidine, cinchonine and cinchonidine. Quinine salts are extensively used as antimalarials. The oldest and most important use of this alkaloid is to treat malarial fever. Major part of world's production of cinchona bark is employed in the manufacture of quinine. Quinidine salts is cardiac dipressent and is used to cure arterial fiberillation. *Cinchona* trees are affected by a member of diseases. The major diseases are caused by fungi (Maiti and Chattopadhyay, 1986).

1. Seedling Blight

Seedling blight of *Cinchona* caused by *Phytophthora* species have plagued growers in many parts of Asia and Africa. A similar disease was found economically important in establishing *Cinchona* plantations in South America. The disease was first observed in Darjeeling district of West Bengal and a species of *Phytophthora* was found to be the causal agent (McRae, 1933). The disease was observed in Guatemala at several locations on seedlings of *C. succirubra* and *C. officinalis* and its different forms. The disease was observed in Puerto Rico on nursery stock of Ledger form of *C. officinalis*.

Symptoms : The disease was found to be destructive to the seedlings in the nursery. A discoloured area is evident in the collar region of the seedlings during the onset of the disease. The discolouration gradually extends until it reaches the cotyledons, which became flaccid and turned downwards. The leaves gradually became yellow, lost their turgidity and many fell down in extreme cases. Discoloured area soon showed rotting which proceeded from the bark to the vascular region and the seedlings gradually drooped downwards and eventually died. Under moist conditions, copious mycelial growth was observed on the rotted tissue.

Causal organism : *Phytophthora palmivora* Butl. The fungus produced moderate aerial growth on the medium. Aerial hyphae are broader than the submerged ones. Sporangia formed sparingly in culture. They are terminal, rarely intercalary, with distinct pedicel, broadly ovate, pearshaped, ellipsodial to spherical with distinct papilla, measuring 17.5 x 58.5 x 9.0 – 30.0 µm, the average being 33.3 x 17.6 µm. Germination may be direct by germ tube under higher temperature or indirect through the production of zoospores at lower temperatures. Each sporangium produces 13-20 zoospores and they are liberated through the papillae (Kheswalla, 1935). Oospores formed has not been found neither on host nor on culture. However, oospore formation has been reported in mixed cultures with other species of *Phytophthora* (McRae, 1932, Kheswalla, 1935).

Mycelium of the fungus is often found in the infected area of bark cortex and wood. The hyphae are both inter and intra cellular. Haustoria are not usually found. Loosely attached sporangia are found on the aerial mycelium. Sporangia on the host usually measure 30-79 x 21.6-45 µm (52 x 44 µm). Optimum temperature for the growth of the fungus was found 24°C. The fungus perpetuates in soil as oospores. The spread is mainly by zoospores through water.

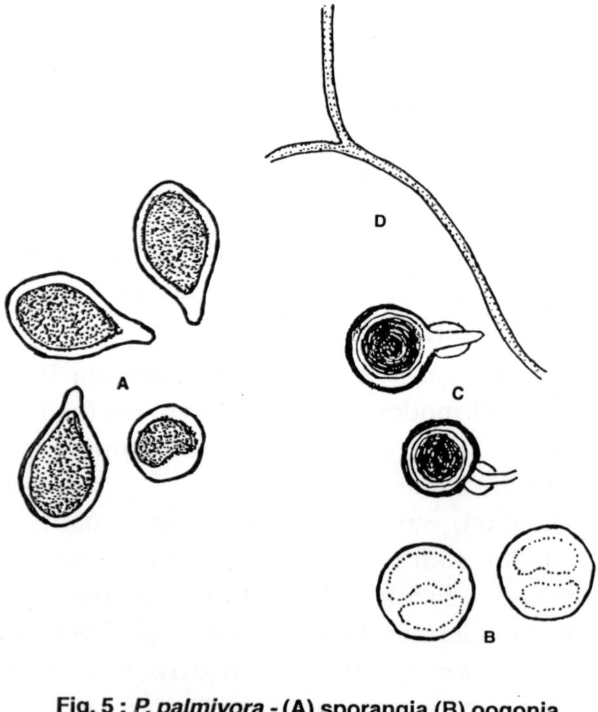

Fig. 5 : *P. palmivora* - (A) sporangia (B) oogonia (C) chlamydospores (D) hyphae

Celino (1934) reported severe blight of *C. calisaya* var. *ledgeriana*, *C. hybrida* and *C. succirubra* caused by *P. faberi* Maubl (Syn : *P. palmivora*). The disease was also observed on Cinchona plants in Taiwan and India (Sawada, 1936, Kheswalla, 1935). The disease affected only seedlings. However, a disease with similar symptoms was observed in Central and South America on seedlings, grafted stock and mature and semi-matured plants. A similar disease was observed in Puerto Rico on seedlings. The infection court seems to be the petiole region of the tender leaves or succulent stem tissue. In early stages the fungus caused brown, necrotic spots with indefinite margins. From initial infections at the base of leaf blades the fungus grew through the entire length of the petiole and the stem. Severely infected seedlings and trees were killed by the pathogen (Crandll and Davis, 1945). The disease was observed in Guatemala at several locations on seedlings of *C. pubesens* Vabl (*C. succirubra*) and *C. officinalis*. The disease was observed in Puerto Rico on *C. officinalis*. The pathogen caused stem cankers and die-back on *Cinchona* species in Colombia.

Control : Attempts have been made to control the disease. In Peru control was apparently obtained by eradicating wilted seedling from the beds. Regular application of copper fungicides along with good sticker could be able to control *Phytophthora*. Selection of resistant high alkaloid containing clones would be the most suitable method of control. Attempts have been made to control the disease by soil fumigation or soil sterilization. In Indonesia effective control was obtained by weekly application of fungicides. Winters (1951) obtained good results in preventing the diseases caused by *Phytophthora* species by (i) application of chloropicrin or DD mixture at a rate of 336 kg/ha., (ii) injecting 2 ml of the chemical at 20 days intervals at 10-12 cm depth or (iii) sprinkling dilute formalin or (iv) drenching with carbamate fungicide. Spraying of the foliage and the base of the stem and drenching the soil with 10% Bordeaux mixture or any other copper fungicide is practiced for the control of the disease.

2. Die-back

Symptoms : Seedlings of *C. officinalis* and some Cinchona hybrids were found to be affected by tip blight disease or die-back. The disease was characterized by necrosis and death of terminal portions of the branches and leaves of young seedlings. The disease was prevalent in Peru (Szkolnik, 1951).

Causal organisms : *Phytophthora parasitica* Dast. The pathogen was isolated from leaf blade, petiole and stem material. Eight day old cultures on corn-meal often produced prominently pappilate sporangia with average size of 30x24 μm on branching sporangiophores 2 days after the plates were flooded with water. This is apparently the first record of the occurrence of the species on Cinchona as well as the first reported *Phytophthora* blight of Cinchona in western hemisphere (Crandall and Davis, 1945). The disease is very severe in Costa Rica where it is referred to top blight (Coster, 1941).

Control : Destruction of dead plants and spraying of Bordeaux mixture have been found useful to control the disease. In Gautemala, control was secured and considerable plants were salvaged by cutting the top of infected grafted stock to well below the dead tip.

3. Pink-disease

The disease was first reported from Darjeeling (Mc Rae, 1930). The disease was found to be present for a long time in West India and Indonesia (Butler, 1918). The disease is believed to cause wide spread damages to

Cinchona plants. *C. ledgeriana* was found to suffer more than *C. succirubra* because of the crowded nature of the foliage.

Symptoms : The disease usually affected small twigs and branches. The leaves were found to lose their colour, gradually turned yellow. The branches also withered rapidly. The affected part is often covered with rose or white crust and somewhat cracked on the underside of the infected branches. The spread of the disease was influenced by moisture. The crust was more pronounced on shaded sides. The pink layer, became ochraceous or white with age. After the pink stage, the spore forming stage which was earlier known as nectar stage of the disease appeared. The extent of damage depended upon the size of the tree. The crust tissue were usually dead. The fungus persisted from one season to another as dormant mycelium formed around canker or in the bark. Humid atmosphere and shady conditions were essential for the establishment of the pathogen.

Causal organism : Corticium salmonicolor Berk & Br (*Syn: Pellicularia salmonicolor* (Berk & Br) Dastur.

The mycelium consists of fine, white, sparsely septate, thin walled hyphae cropping over the surface of the bark, either forming white sheets or remaining thread like. Hyphae later aggregate into dense coils to form nodules chiefly in the lenticle. The neighbourhood of the nodules, the cells of the host tissue are killed and turned brown. This appears to be the first stage of attack.

Fruiting body extending several cm over surface of bark, resupinate, membranaceous, often about 500 µm thick, smooth, salmon pink when fresh fading to light cream or whitish when dry. All hyphae without clamps, hyaline, smooth, distinct. Basal hyphae 6-10 µm diam., cells 30-150 µm long, walls up to 1.5 µm thick, sparsely branched, branching usually at a fairly wide angel.

Hymenial branches narrower, short celled, thin walled and more richly branched than basal hyphae. Basidial stage when formed, is resupinate made up a lose layer of interwoven hyphae, densely packed basidia. Basidia obovoid to broadly clavate when young, narrowly clavate to cylindrical when mature, thin-walled, smooth, 30-55 x 5-10 μm with 4 slightly inwardly-curved sterigmata approximately 4-6 x 1-5-2 μm. Spores broadly ellipsoidal with prominent apiculus, thin-walled smooth, not amyloid, dextrinoid or cyanophilous 10-13 x 6-9 μm. Sporodochia of conidial state discoid, erumpent or superficial on bark, forming orange-red pustules of conidiogenous cells. These fragment by separation at the septa to form hyaline thin-walled unicellular ellipsoid conidia 10-19 (13) x 6-12 (8.5) μm. The spores are individually hyaline, collectively pink. Under artificial conditions, the fungus forms only sterile creeping mycelium often with nodular form. No fruiting bodies are formed in culture.

Control : Only some cultural practices and prophylatic treatment might be useful for reducing the losses caused by the disease. Less favourable condition for the establishment of the disease can be created by providing less humid atmosphere. Free circulation of air, reduction of shade, thin planting and good drainage. Cutting of disease affected branches and their destruction by burning might also help to reduce disease incidence. Prophylatic spray of 1% Bordeaux mixture has been recommended for the pink disease of rubber (Butler, 1918). However, prophylatic spray recommended in other cases might be useful in controlling the disease on cinchona.

4. Canker

Two distinct bark disease of Cinchona, called stripe canker and girdle canker have been reported to cause

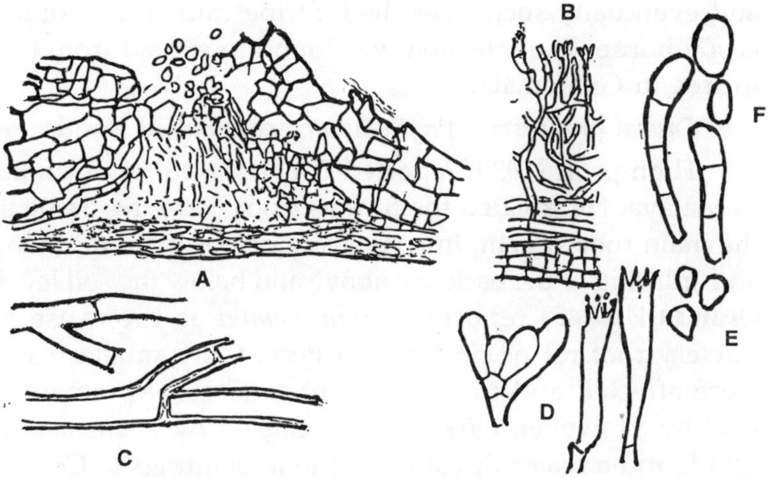

Fig. 6 : *C. salmonicolor* - (A) nectar state (B) vertical section of fruiting body on surface of bark (C) basal hyphae (D) young and mature basidia (E) basidiospores (F) conidiogenous cells and mature conidia

serious losses to plantings in Guatemala. Stripe canker is found in the rootstock and scion of practically all clones, however, girdle canker appeared to be localized just above the union in the scion of some selections and hybrids (Darley and Flores, 1951). Bark canker of cinchona discribed from East Indies and West Java might probably be the strip canker.

(a) Stripe canker : Infection apparently originated in the roots and advanced upward through the union and into the stem of the tree. The disease is characterized by vertical, linear, slightly sunken stripes of dead and dying inner bark. The stripe varied in width and length and reached to the full length of the tree in later stages. There might be several infection courts in roots giving rise to several stripes on the stem. In some instance multiple stripes developed on the stem. As the disease spread upwards, droplets of dark, sticky exudate appeared on the surface of infected bark. The leaves of infected trees in some clones became yellow when several stripes developed

and eventually such trees died. Stripe canker apparently is soil-borne. The infection was found to spread from tree to tree in Guatemala.

Causal organism : Phytophthora cinnamomi Rands.

Thompson (1939) reported *P. cinnamomi* on cinchona in Malaya. He isolated the fungus from decaying tissue in the main root system. In some trees he observed decaying and splitting of the bark just above and below the soil level. Crandall (1947) reported *P. cinnamomi* as the cause of nursery root rot of cinchona in Peru. Only smaller roots were affected and the larger roots and crown remained healthy. However, bark disease, caused by *P. cinnamomi* was found a major threat to cinchona plantings in Central Africa. The disease was also found to occur in India on *C. succirubra* on *C. ledgeriana* (Ramakrishnan, 1951).

(b) Girdle canker : The girdle canker girdles the tree. The bark of the scion above the graft union is killed and became sunken in a horizontal band. The sunken appearance is accentuated by inrolling of callus tissue above and below the dead area. The canker may spread upto the stem of the scion and no true infection was found to go below the graft union into the root stock. Leaves turned yellow and there was a gradual die-back of twigs and branches, culminating eventually in the death of entire tree. It was reported that the infection took place through the leaves and petioles of small shoots at the base of the scion and advanced into the bark of the main stem where girdling occurred. In some cases dead shoots remained attached to the scion at the site of girdle lesion. In other cases leaves and petioles of small shoots were found to wilt and die (Darley and Flores, 1951).

Causal organism : Phytophthora parasitica Dastur.

Control : Destruction of diseased plants and spraying the plants with fungicides as a prophylatic measure are the only control measures for both the canker diseases.

5. Damping-off

Damping-off of *Cinchona* seedlings and wilting of sprouts of vegetatively propagated nurseries have been reported from South India (Ramakrishnan, 1949).

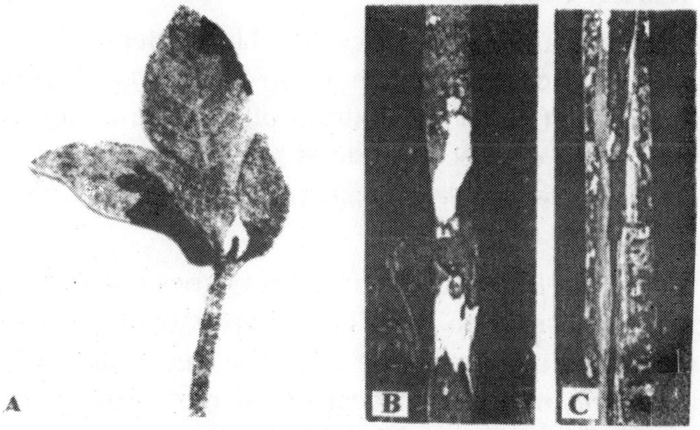

Fig. 7 : Cinchona diseases (A) die-back caused by *P. parasitica* (B) stripe canker caused by *P. cinnamomi* (C) girdle canker caused by *P. parasitica*

Symptoms : Roots of infected seedlings or sprouts showed rotting and water soaked lesions appeared at the base below soil level. One to three year old plants were also affected. The infected plants showed reddening of leaves which drooped down and ultimately defoliated. Large number of roots of such plants were blackened and died. The cortex of the roots easily sloughed off. Hyphae were present in the cortex and sometimes in xylem vessels.

Causal organism : *Pythium vexans* de Bary. Hyphae without septa. Zoosporangia not formed except on germination of oospores. Oogonia smooth, spherical, light yellow to brown, sessile, antheridia single, club shaped, rising close to the oogonium from the same hyphae. Oospore single, spherical, wall thin, light yellow to brown, germination by hyphae or zoospores. The fungus survived in soil as oospores and the spread took place through zoospores.

Control : Some of the control measures used against diseases caused by *Pythium* species can be adopted. However, no specific control measure for this disease has been recommended.

6. Brown Root-rot

The disease was first described by Butler (1918) on tea. The occurrence of this disease on *Cinchona* was reported by Sundram (1928). The extend of damage is not known although the disease is wide spread.

Causal organism : *Fomes lamaoensis* (Murr) Sacc & Trott.

Control : Removal of diseased bushes and old stumps would be useful to restrict the spread of the disease. Application of quick-lime near the decaying bushes or stumps are practiced to destroy all remnants of affected roots. This.practice might minimize the chances of spread of the disease.

7. Minor Diseases

(a) Damping-off : Damping-off of seedlings was commonly observed in over crowded nurseries particularly at the lower elevation. The disease was caused by *Macrophomina phaseoli* (Mauld) Ashby (Winters, 1950). Removal of affected plants and excess of shade, restricting watering and application of copper fungicide were recommended for control. Treating the seed beds with chloropcrin before sowing and covering the soil with sphagenum moss is helpful in preventing the disease.

(b) Root and Collar-rot : Seedling in the nursery were found to be affected by root-rot and collar-rot. Colar-rot was also observed in young trees. The disease was reported to be caused by *Sclerotium rolfsii* Sacc. Destruction of dead plants and earthing up the trees were found to help in reducing the spread of the disease.

3
COLEUS

Coleus forskohlii (Wild) Briq. is an Indian medicinal plant which was very little known until recently, has now been raised to an internationally important medicinal plant because of the research efforts on this plant during the last few years. It is a perennial aromatic herb growing wild from Simla eastwards to Nepal, in the hills of Bihar, Gujarat and Peninsular India. The plant is cultivated in Maharashtra and Gujarat for edible roots which are often used as pickles (Abraham *et.al.*, 1988).

The plant is distributed over the subtropics, warm atmosphere climatic zone on the mountains of India, Nepal, Sri Lanka, Africa, Burma and Thailand. The pharmacological studies of *C. forskohlii* revealed cardiovascular property of the root extracts. This led to the isolation of a diterpene, forskolin. Forskolin has been reported to possess a large number of biological properties such as antihypertensive, bronchospasmolytic, antithrombotic, platelet aggregation inhibition, antiglaucoma and adenylatecyclase stimulation. The drug is claimed to improve appettite, facilitate digestion, increase vitality and is useful in anaemia, inflammation, fever, dysentery, chronic abdominal problems, etc. (De Souza, 1991). Forskolin has been developed as a hypotensive and cardiotonic drug. *Coleus forskohlii* is being cultivated to a limited extent for root tuber in Gujarat, Maharashtra and Karnataka in India. The plant is reported to be affected by only a few diseases till now.

1. Leaf Blight

Severe leaf infection of C. *forskohlii* cultivated in the experimental plantations has been reported during cool, cloudy and rainy weather.

Symptoms : Symptoms consisted of water soaked leaf spots that increased rapidily in size and became light and then turned to brown in colour. The spots coalesced resulting in blight symptoms. Severe infection caused defoliation and death of the plants (Shukla *et.al.*, 1993).

Causal organism : *Rhizoctonia solani* Kuhn.

2. Root-knot

Coleus forskohlii is reported to be affected by root-gall or root-knot disease. This is the most important disease of this crop reported till now. Nematode infected plants though stunted appear as luxuriant as the normal plants. Heavy infection of root-knot nematode was observed in the farms in Gujarat (Patel *et.al.*, 1987). The disease was found to affect the plants in the third month after planting.

Symptoms : The symptoms consist of stunting, wilting of leaves and the basal part of the stem turned brownish-black. The diseased roots are totally damaged. The infection caused yellow patches in the plantations. Due to severe galling tuber formation was reduced nearly 65 per cent in field conditions (Rajendran and Vadivelu, 1991).

Causal organism : Meloidogyne incognita (Kofoid & White) Chitwood.

Control : Attempts have been made to control the disease by biological control methods (Sivakumar and Vidhyasekharan, 1990). However, crop rotation and use of suitable nematocides would be beneficial to minimize the loss of yield.

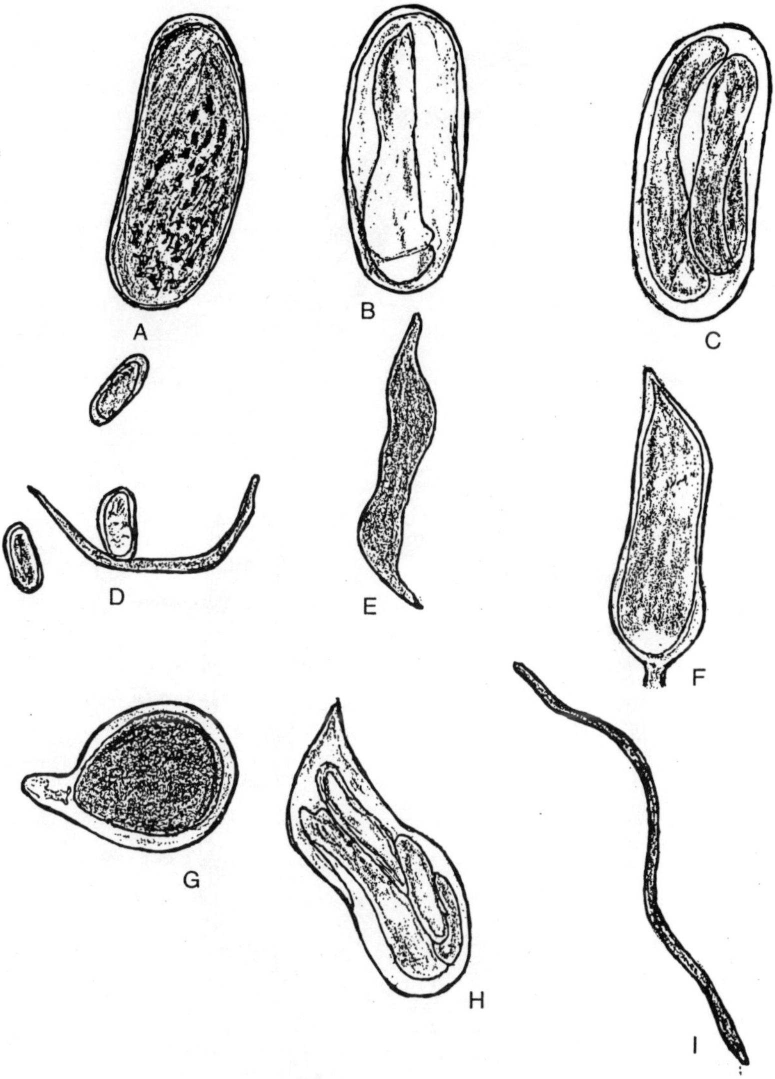

Fig. 8 : Development stages of *M. incognita* (A) undifferentiated egg (B) first stage larva (C) second stage larva (D) free living second stage infectious larva (E) sexually differentiated second stage larva (F) third stage larva (G) adult female (H) adult male just after fourth moult (I) adult male (Courtesy of Dr. P.C. Trivedi Dept. of Botany, University of Rajasthan)

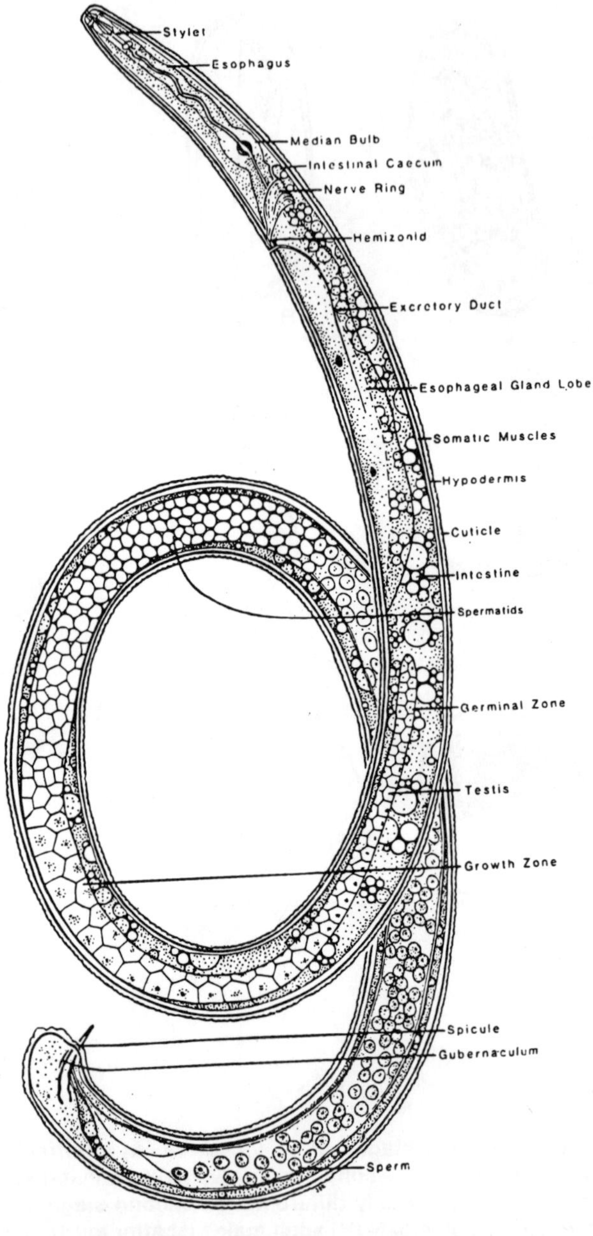

Fig. 9 : Morphology of male root-knot nematode - *M. incognita*
(Courtesy of Dr. P.C. Trivedi Dept. of Botany, University of Rajasthan)

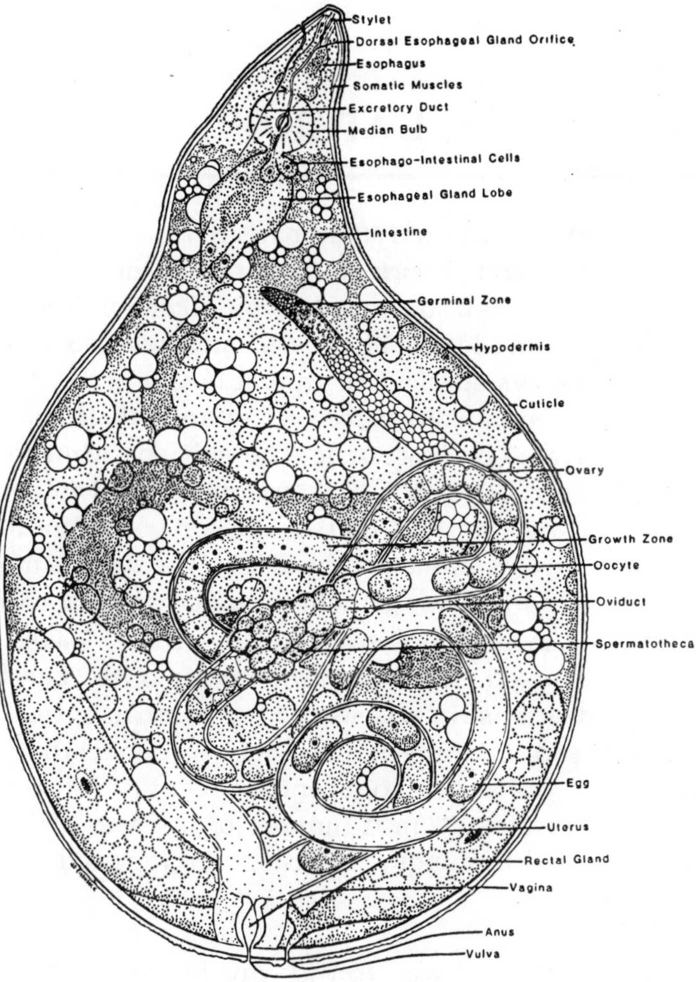

Fig. 10 : Morphology of female root-knot nematode - *M. incognita*
(Courtesy of Dr. P.C. Trivedi Dept. of Botany, University of Rajasthan)

4
DATURA

Various species of *Datura* namely *D. innoxia* Mill. *D. stramonium* L. and *D. metel* L. are used in medicine, both as crude as well as a source of tropane alkaloids. The seeds of *D. innoxia* and leaves of *D. metel* are used as source of hyoscine. *Datura* species are annual bushy herbs. *Datura* is not an economical source of tropane alkaloids. It is rarely cultivated on large scale. The only species which is still used in crude form is *D. stramonium* and is cultivated in Europe and South America. Major constituents of *Datura* are hyoscyamine and hyoscine. The drug is mostly used in crude form as anticholinergic agent in case of asthma and intestinal disorders. *Datura* seeds, leaves and roots are used in insanity, fever with cerebral complications, skin diseases and as antiseptic. The alkaloid, scopolamine is used as a preanaesthetic in surgery, in ophthalmology and prevention of motion sickness (Husain, 1993). A number of diseases of *Datura* species caused by fungi and viruses are reported.

1. Leaf Spot

The disease was found on leaves of *Datura stramonium, D. metel* and *D. innoxia*. A large number of plants growing in the experimental plantations were found to suffer by the disease.

Symptoms : The infection caused severe defoliation causing considerable economic loss (Ganguly and Pandotra, 1962). Spots are characteristically dark-brown, round to oval or slightly irregular, coalescing and forming large necrotic area.

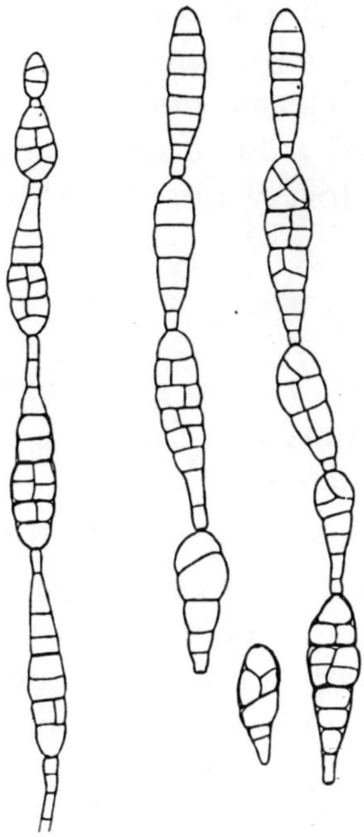

Fig. 11 : *A. tenuissima* – conidia in chains

Causal organism : Alternaria tenuissima (Fr) Wiltshire. Conidophore simple, moderate length chain of 5-10 or more conidia, significant number of them are long and narrow. Initial chain may remain simple, but commonly it produces one or a few lateral branches of a few conidia. Conidia in chain often have a narrow-tapered upper half. Conidia in the distal part of a chain usually are ovoid or ellipsoid without a narrow taper in the upper half, each conidium produces a short apical secondary conidiophore of 1-2 cells. Narrow conidia have only transverse septa. Wider conidia have both trans-septa (5-8) and a few longitudinal or oblique septa in the broadest segments of the spore body. Only, one or two of the largest conidia in a chain in culture have constricting transverse septum which is a striking feature of field conidia. Conidia having only trans-septa reach a size approximately 32-45 x 11-13 µm, ovoid muriformally septate conidia approximately 32-45 x 14-18 µm, obclavate muriformally septate conidia approximately 40-60 x 16-18 µm. Conidia are medium gold-brown and closely obscurely to conspicuously punctulate.

2. Leaf Blight

Datura innoxia growing in experimental and commercial plantations was found to suffer from a leaf blight disease.

Symptoms : Early infection of the disease appeared as water soaked circular spots on the leaves. In later stages the spots coalesced, became dull yellow and turned light brown due to the death of infected tissue. Concentric rings appeared on the dead tissue of old spots. A single spct on a leaf caused curling of the entire leaf in advance sta;;e of infection. Wilting of the entire branch occurred when two or three leaves of a branch were affected. The leaves of affected branch curled and this was followed by death and defoliation of the plants. Older leaves were more suncepticable as compared to younger ones (Janardhanan and Husain, 1972).

Causal organism : Alternaria alternata (Fr) Keissler. The hyphae are branched, septate and dark brown in colour. The conidia are borne on conidiophores in chains, dark brown in colour. Sporulation pattern comprises a single suberect conidiophore and an apical cluster of branching chain of small conidia separated by short secondary conidiophores. The primary conidiophore is comparatively short approximately 40-70 x 3-4 µm, it remains simple or may become 1-3 branched or geniculate with corresponding number of primary conidial chains. Single

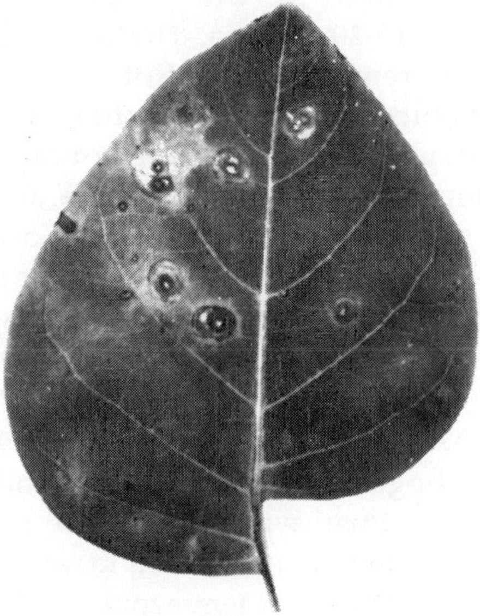

Fig. 12 : Symptoms of leaf blight of *D. innoxia* caused by *A. alternata*

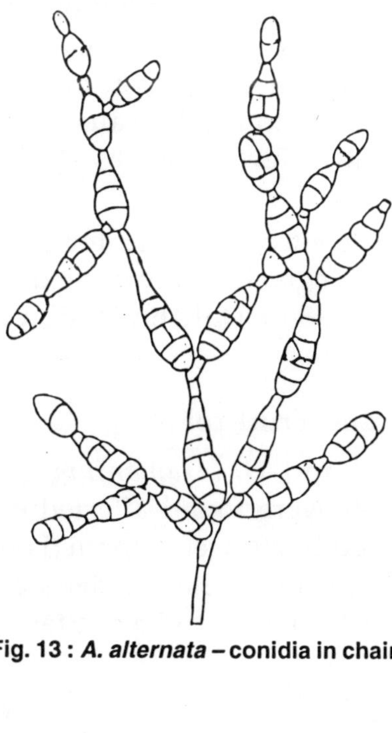

Fig. 13 : *A. alternata* – conidia in chains

chains of conidia in the branching head have approximately 15-20 conidia. The first 1-2 conidia in a chain usually remain long-elliptical as they mature, conidia produced later in the chain become ovoid, elloipsoid or subsphaeroid. Initial elliptical conidia are 14-52 x 8-16 μm with 4-7 transverse septa and a few or no longisepta, subsequent spores are 7-40 x 5-12 μm with 1-7 transepta-(commonly 3) and very few or no longisepta. The conidia are dark brown in colour. They became pale yellowish to golden brown after a few days in lactic acid mounts, wall ornamentation is densely punctulate, granular to variously verrucose as conidia mature.

The pathogen is reported to produce a toxic metabolite. The toxin was found to be responsible for chlorosis and yellowing of infected leaves. The toxin was isolated and identified as tenuazonic acid (Janardhanan and Husain, 1975, 1983). The toxin showed significant phytotoxic activity against a number of plants. The toxin was reported to induce significant reduction in chlorophyll and protein contents in infected leaves. This activity is suggested to be the cause of chlorosis and necrosis found in infected leaves (Janardhanan and Husain, 1984).

Control : No control measure for the disease is reported. However, fungicidal spray using dithiocarbamates, such as Dithane Z-78 or Dithane M-45 would be useful to control the disease.

3. Leaf Blight and Fruit-rot

Datura metel and *D. stramonium* growing in the experimental plots were found affected by this disease. Leaf blight and pod blight were reported on *D. metel* from Israel (Halfon-Meiri, 1973). Similar disease was found on *D. stramonium* in Lucknow, India (Sattar *et.al.*, 1986).

Synrtoms : The infection was first observed on leaves as small necrotic spots. The infection was later spread to the fruits resulting in fruit blight and rot. The mycelium penetrated beneth the seed-coat in most infected seeds.

Causal organisms : *Alternaria crassa* (Sacc) Rands. Conidiophores arise single or in groups, straight or flexuosus, sometimes geniculate, septate, pale or pale brown up to 90 µm long, 7-10 µm thick with one to several scars. Conidia usually solitary, occasionally in very short chains, obclavate, rostrate, beak generally exceeding the length of the body of the spore, pale brown, smooth 120-440 (250) x 15-40 (22) µm in size, 7-10 transverse and usually several longitudinal septa, beak pale brown, septate, not branched 4-8 µm thick at the base, tapering to 2-2.5 µm.

The fungus was reported to produce a phytotoxic metabolite *in vitro*. The metabolite was isolated and

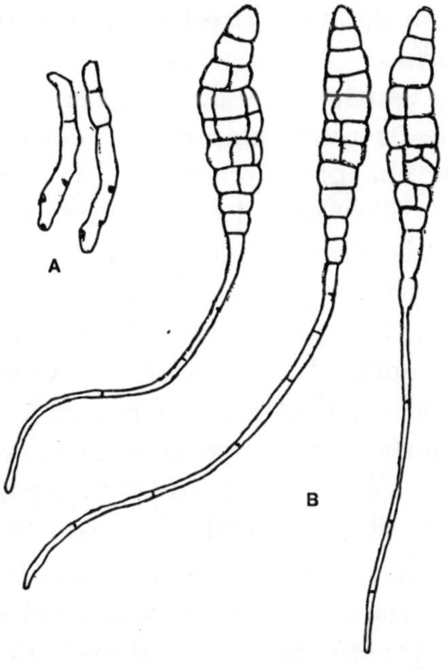

Fig. 14 : *A. crassa* – (A) conidiophores (B) conidia

identified as tenuazonic acid (Sattar *et.al.*, 1986). Tenuazonic acid induced typical necrosis on *D. stramonium* leaves.

Control : Excellent control of the fungus was achieved by disinfection with Thiram suspension. Seed treatment with organo-mercurial dust did not give efficient control of the fungus (Halfon-Meir, 1973).

4. Root-rot

Two root diseases of *D. innoxia* have been reported. Infected plants showed yellowing, gradual wilting resulting in the death of plants. Nearly 15-20 percent plants growing in experimental plantations were found to be affected by the disease (Thakur and Sastry, 1970).

Causal organisms : *Sclerotium rolfsii* Sacc. Colonies on potato dextrose agar white with narrow mycelial strands, sclerotia developed on the surface. The sclerotia nearly spherical, 1-2 μm dia. when fresh with smooth or shallow pitted shiny surface. Cells of primary hyphae at advancing edge of colony usually 4.5-9 μm wide and up to 350 μm long with one or more clamp connections at septa. Sclerotia show sharply diferentiated rind with evenly thickened walls. Cortex and medulla contain vesicles of reserve materials. The hymenium is described on agar medium as white to ochraceous stromata sparse or aggregated in irregular masses. Basidia clavate, basidiospores smooth, hyaline, globose-pyriform, 4.5-6.75 x 3.5-4.5 μm. On the host plants white mycelium spread over near soil surface. Appressoria develop as swollen tips of short branches behind the advancing edge. Sclerotia usually develop after the death the host plants.

Control : Usual control measures include disinfection of planting materials, adjustment of soil pH and fertilizer regime. Cultural methods, such as deep burial of infected crop residue and crop rotation are often beneficial. Use of soil fumigants such as formalin, methylbromide are also beneficial. Pentachlobenzene is considered to be useful to control the fungus.

Another root and foot-rot of *D. innoxia* showing almost similar symptoms was observed in the experimental plantations (Thakur, 1974). The disease affected plants of all ages, more destructive on young plants. Seedlings showed damping-off and were killed within weeks. In matured plants older leaves showed yellowing. As the disease advanced, severe rotting occurred leading to death and disintegration of plants.

Causal organism : Corticium solani (Perill & Delacr) Bourd & Glaz.

5. Distortion Mosaic

The virus caused severe systemic mosaic with puckering and leaf distortion in *D. stramonium.* The disease was reported to be caused by a strain of cucumber mosaic virus (Singh, 1980, El-Hammady *et.al.*, 1977). This disease was also reported on *D. innoxia*. The main symptoms were yellowing of veins followed by slight inward rolling and distortion of leaves. The virus was identified as Datura virus-3 or Datura virus-3A (Sastry *et.al.*, 1977, Capoor and Verma, 1952). Symptoms of systemic mottling leaf distortion and vein banding occur in *D. stramonium*. The virus is a flexuosus filamentous particle and is single stranded RNA and identified as Tobacco etch virus.

Previously undescribed two rhabdo-virus was isolated from Queensland from *D. stramonium* with symptoms of vein yellowing, leaf distortion and reduced leaf size (Thomas and Dietzgen, 1991). The virus was named as Datura yellow vein virus (DYVV) and was graft transmitted to several solanaceous hosts. The virus was not transmitted mechanically or by vectors. The virus was isolated and the serological relationship studied. The virus was described as a new rhabdovirus.

6. Virus Wilt

Early symptoms of the disease on *D. stramonium, D. innoxia* and *D. metel* were vein clearing followed by necrosis which spread over conducting elements of leaf stalk and stem, resulting in wilting of leaves and whole plants. The virus was transmitted non-persistently by *Myzus persicae*. No identification of the virus is known (Kovachevski, 1974).

7. Little Leaf

The infected plants showed retarded growth. The leaves became smaller and pale in colour. Infected plants flowered rarely and leaves were small crowded at internodes and apex of the branches. The infection was observed on *D. metel*. The virus was graft transmissable to *D. innoxia* and *D. stramonium* apart from other plants (Sastry *et.al.*, 1977).

8. Mosaic

A number of mosaic diseases have been reported on *Datura* species. Symptoms showed alternatively dark and light green patches, varying in size and shape on leaf lamina and growth was retarded. The symptoms were similar to Tobacco mosaic virus (TMV). Electron microscopic studies showed straight, rod-like particles similar to TMV (Khotin *et.al.*, 1973). Piccirillo and Caponigro (1992) also found a TMV strain causing systemic infection on *D. metel*. Callose deposition during hypersensetive reaction on *D. stramonium* infected with TMV was observed. Callose formation probably restricted the movement of the virus (Conti *et.al.*, 1983).

Two sap transmissible, aphid-borne viruses infecting *D. metel* and *D. innoxia* causing mosaiç symptoms were reported from Akola, India (Gahukar and Patil, 1991). Naturally infected plants showed severe mosaic mottling accompanied with blistering, distortion and various leaf deformities. The leaf lamina of apical leaves was completely supressed, exhibiting shoe-string appearance. The virus was named as *Datura metel* mosaic virus (DMMV) and *Datura innoxia* mosaic virus (DIMV). Based on the serology the virus was identified as a strain of a potty virus, Datura distortion mosaic virus.

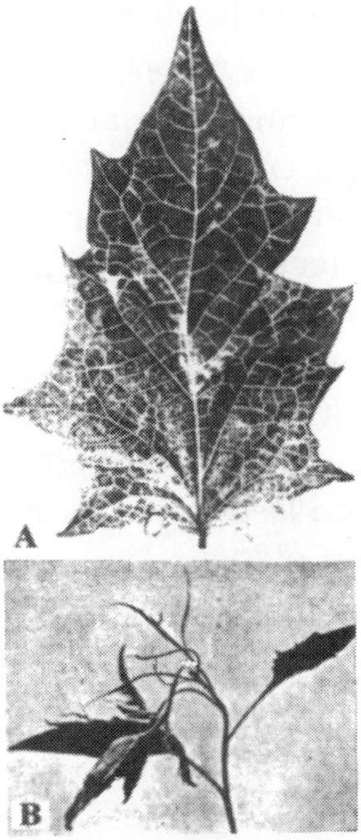

Fig. 15 : (A) *D. stramonium* infected with mosaic virus (B) *D. metel* showing symptoms of leaf distortion and mosaic

A virus disease producing symptoms of vein clearing, mosaic, leaf puckering, distortion and filiform leaves on *D. metel* growing in waste land was reported from Andhra

Pradesh, India. The virus was sap transmitted non-persistently by insects. Cytoplasmic cylindrical inclusions in epidermal cells of infected *D. metel* leaves were observed under light microscope. The partially purified preparations contained flexuosus filamentous virus particles. The causal virus was identified as a potyvirus (Prasanna, 1996).

A potyvirus was also isolated from *D. stramonium* in Yemen. It was transmitted mechanically and by *Myzus persicae* in a non-persistant manner. The virus particle was flexuosus rod-shaped. The virus showed distinct serological relationship to pepper veinal mottle potyvirus (PVMV) and potato Y potyvirus. The virus was tentatively named tomato mild mottle virus (Walkey, 1994).

A mosaic disease of *D. metel* causing stunted growth, reduction in leaf size and light and dark green areas on leaf blade with blighter like patches was reported from India. Mechanical transmission of the virus was successful and other hosts infected were *D. stramonium, Petunia hybrida* and *Nicotiana plumbaginifolia*. The name Datura virus-3B was proposed (Yaraguntaiah and Govindu, 1972).

Sastry *et.al.,* (1977) reported a mosaic disease of *D. innoxia*. The mosaic infected plants showed retarded growth and produced lesser number of flowers and fruits compared to healthy plants.

5
DIGITALIS

Digitalis was used in folk medicine in England as early as tenth century. The plant is a native of British Island and Western Europe. *Digitalis purpurea* L. is a biennial (annual in subtropic) herbaceous plant. It is cultivated for medicinal purposes in England, Germany, Hungary, USA and Russia. Powdered leaf extract as well as glycosides isolated from *D. purpurea* are used in medicine for various ailments. Its main effect is on cardiovascular system. Digitalis products are cardiotonics, increase contractibility of heart and improve tone of the heart muscles. Two main digitalis glycosides used in medicine are digitoxin and gitalin. Digitoxin is used to improve tone of cardiac muscles and gitalin is employed in congestive heart failure. *Digitalis lanata* Ehrh. is related to *D. purpurea*. During the last 20 years glycosides from *D. lanata* are used. *Digitalis lanata* is native of Southern and Central Europe. The plant is cultivated in Switzerland, the Netherlands, Russia, Germany and UK. In India, *Digitalis* species are cultivated in Nilgiri Hills, Darjeeling, Kashmir valley, Himachal Pradesh and hills of Uttar Pradesh. *Digitalis lanata* is annual, biennial or perennial herb. Nearly 70 glycosides have been reported from the leaves of *D. lanata*, of these, lanatoside C and digoxin are most important glycosides used in medicine. Both lanatoside C and digoxin are most commonly used drug in congestive heart failure and various other heart ailments (Husain, 1993). *Digitalis* species have been reported to be affected by a number of diseases caused by fungi and viruses.

1. Anthracnose

This disease has been reported from USA, UK, Japan, Czechoslovakia and other European countries and Asia (Goto 1938). *Digitalis purpurea*, the principal species grown in United States has not been severally affected by the disease. However, *D. lanata* was known to be affected with anthracnose disease in USA. The disease caused almost complete devastation in some areas (Thomas, 1951).

Symptoms : Symptoms are consisted of purplish-brown, circular or angular spots, 1 to 4 µm in diameter on the leaf surfaces; small, sunken, fusiform lesions occur on veins and petioles. Numerous dark brown setae are produced in the black, pulvirate acervuli . A large number of nerotic patches appear in the later stages and these necrotic spots coalesced leading to the death of the leaves. The spread of the disease has been reported through conidia. The pathogen is known to be seed borne and it easily spread in the seed beds. Lesions often do not appear on the first leaves of seedlings grown in outdoor seed beds before they are transplanted to the field. Infection becomes general and severe by late summer or early fall. Severly affected plants are killed before the herb is ready for harvest. This resulted in heavy loss (Thomas, 1951). The disease caused considerable damage to *D. lanata* in commercial plantings. All five species namely, *D. sibirica* Lindl., *D. purpurea*, *D. ambigua* Murr., *D. ferruginea* L. and *D. lanata* tested were susceptible to the disease, among them *D. ferruginea* and *D. lanata* were the most susceptible.

Causal organism : *Colletotrichum fuscum* Laub.

Control : The anthracnose disease could be avoided by using disease free seeds. The use of noninfested seeds gave complete freedom from disease. Hot water treatment at 55°C for 15 min. was found to control the organism. Marked reduction in germination usually resulted from treatments longer than 15 min. Seed treatment with a number of fungicides were found to be injurious. Spraying of the crops with 0.5% Bordeaux mixture was found beneficial. Crop rotation and field sanitation also found useful to check the disease (Thomas, 1951).

2. Leaf-spot

Digitalis purpurea and *D. lanata* were reported to be affected by a number of leaf spot diseases. However, two of them were considered economically important.

Symptoms : The disease appeared on leaves as circular spots with purple margin and later the spots became irregular and necrotic with numerous pycnidia in stroma. The fungus has been reported to cause more damage at the cotyledonery stage of the seedlings as also on young plants. Perpetuation of the disease has been known through pycnidia, stroma and partly as mycelium in the necrotic tissue. The disease is externally seed borne (Kowalski, 1968). The disease has been known to occur in Yugoslavia, UK and Japan.

Causal organism : *Septoria digitalis* Pass

Six morphologically distinct forms of *S. digitalis* were isolated from *D. lanata.* The isolates differed in pathogenicity probably indicating the existence of physiologic races. Of the *Digitalis* species tested *D. lanata* was most susceptible and *D. purpurea* was the most resistant (Grzybowska, 1976). The infection also reduced the active principle in *D. lanata* leaves (Dobos, 1988).

Control : Five fungicides were tested for the control of the disease Tilt (propiconazole) at 0.5 lit/ha gave the best protection against the disease (Dobos, 1988).

A leaf spot disease resembling symptoms caused by *Septoria* has been reported from Canada, Belgium, USA and UK. The disease was caused by *Phyllosticta digitalis* Bill. Use of seeds from disease free area for raising the crop, spraying of fungicides such as Bordeaux mixture (0.5-2%) Captan (0.2%) and Zeneb (0.2%) was recommended for the control of the disease (Sastry *et.al.*, 1977).

3. Viral Diseases

A number of viruses have been reported to infect *Digitalis*. Tobacco mosaic virus (TMV) Cucumber mosaic virus (CMV) Tobacco ring spot virus (TRSV) have been reported on *Digitalis* species. Occurrence of beet curly top (BCTV) and broad been wild virus (BWV) have also been occasionally reported. Sastry (1972) found strains of cucumber mosaic virus (CMV) and petunia distortion strains of tobacco mosaic virus causing mosaic symptoms under field conditions (Sastry *et.al.*, 1977).

Ribgrass mosaic virus (RMV) was found to cause mosaic symptoms on *D. lanata* in Germany (Schumann, 1963). The disease caused systemic chlorotic mottling and ring-like marking, chlorotic streak along the veins and slight twisting of the petioles. This is a RNA containing virus with rod-shaped particles, 18 nm wide and 300 nm long. It is found in several wild plant species, occurs in high concentration in sap, is very stable and readily transmitted by inoculation of sap. No vector is known. The virus is widely distributed and reported from Asia, Europe, North America and USSR. Different types of cytoplasmic inclusions were observed in ultrathin sections of *D. purpurea* systemically infected with 3 different strains of RMV. Tissue from uninfected plants did not contain such inclusions. Most common were rounded plates consisting of layers of aligned virus particles 300 nm long. A novel type of inclusion were the abundant spiral aggregates found in *D. purpurea* systemically infected with a strain of RMV. The virus particles were arranged in a circular manner around a centre. The orientation of the particles changes in such a way that virus being 30 nm apart are cut in the longitudinal and in the transverse direction respectively (Ernwein and Wetter, 1987).

6
DIOSCOREA

Rhizomes of *Dioscorea* species are the source of steroidal sapogenin, diosgenin. Diosgenin itself is not a medicinal product, but it is one of the most important raw materials used for the synthesis of steroidal drugs which include corticosteriods, sex hormones, oral contraceptives and anabolic steroides. Although, *Dioscorea* species were used in folk medicine for various diseases, their use as a source of diosgenin was discovered only recently. The use of steroidal hormones in medicine was known for a very long time. Its use was restricted to sex hormones. The important steroidal compounds as therapeutic agents for a wide variety of diseases realised only after the discovery of the use of corticosteroids as antiarthritic and antiinflammatory agents in 1948. The value of these compounds increased further with the discovery of their use as antifertility agent in 1954. Because of these, there was an unprecedented increase in the demand of steroids for health and family planning programmes all over the world. There are more than 15 species of *Dioscorea,* which are reported to contain appreciable amount of diosgenin, occurring in Asia, Africa, Europe, China and South America. Of these species *D. composita* Hensel, *D. floribunda* Mart and Gal from Central and South America and *D. deltoidea* Wall from India are most important. *Dioscorea* are perennial climbing herbs with tubers and rhizomes. Although, *Dioscorea* rhizome contain a variety of chemical substances, the most important constituents are group of saponins which yield sapogenins on hydrolysis. Important sapogenins found in various species of *Dioscorea* are diosgenin, yamogenin, botogenin and kryptogenin. Corticosteroids in the form of cortisones and hydrocortisones are used for treatment of rheumatism, arthritis, rheumatic fever, etc. Both male and female hormones such as testosterone and progestrone are synthesised from diosgenin (Husain, 1993).

Medicinal *Dioscorea* species namely *D. deltoidea, D. floribunda* and *D. composita* are cultivated in many parts of the world. They are reported to be affected by a number of diseases. Leaf spots and tuber rots caused by fungi and mosaic disease caused by virus are the major diseases of these plants.

1. Rust

Symptoms : The rust infection is observed during the months of October-November on *D. deltoidae*. The symptoms consisted of minute scattered pustules of the fungus on the leaf surface. Both uredal and telial stages of the fungus were observed on infected plants. Severe infection resulted in leaf fall (Ganguly and Pandotra, 1962).

Causal organism : *Puccinia dioscorea* Kom.

2. Leaf Spots

Symptoms : *Dioscorea deltoidae* is found to be affected by a leaf spot disease. The symptoms are characterized by numerous scattered spots on the leaves. The spots are irregularly angular, dark brown in colour with indefinite margins (Ganguly and Pandotra 1963). Severe infection caused premature defoliation.

Causal organism : *Cercospora dioscorea* Ellis & Mart. Conidiophores in dense fascicles (upto 40 conidiophores in a fascicle), light brown, septate, unbranched, straight, rarely curved, geniculations rare, 19.6-39.3 x 3.6-4.9 μm. Conidia catenate, cylindrical to narrowly obclavate, truncate at the base 20.9-51.6 x 3.6-7.3 μm (Ganguly and Pandotra 1963).

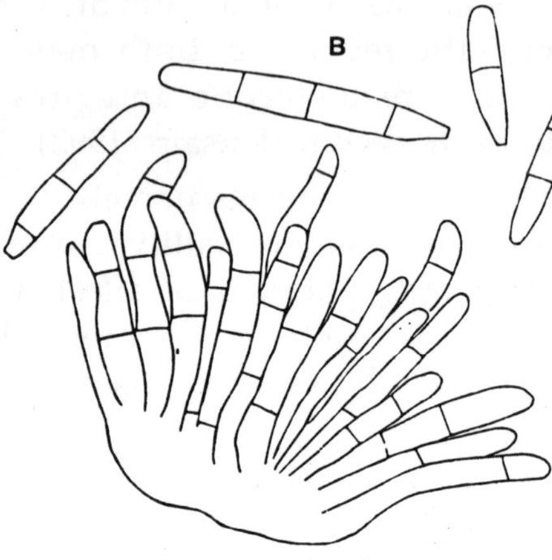

Fig. 16 : *C. dioscorea* – conidiophore and conidia (A) conidophore (B) conidia

Dioscorea floribunda is also found to be affected by a leaf-spot disease. The seedlings are often heavily infected.

Symptoms : The fungus produced circular spots which are surrounded by dark border. The spots enlarged into irregular size. Abundant spores are produced on the infected leaves. Under humid conditions the disease was found to spread through mycelia (Koch, 1964). This resulted in severe disease incidence.

Causal organism : The fungus was identified as a species of *Helminthosporium* (Koch, 1964). The spores were 70-100 μm long, 14-16 μm wide with 5-10 septate and germinate bipolar manner. The spores resembled very much to the spores of *Helminthosporium sacchari* Butler according to the description by Cook (1929).

Control : The best control method was the destruction of all infected leaves as soon as spots appeared. Application of Maneb (manganese ethylene bisdithiocarbamate) twice a week to young seedlings was found to control the disease.

Dioscorea composita was also found to be infected with a leaf spot disease.

Symptoms : The disease was observed in the seedling stage in the nurseries during the months of February-March in Goa (India). The damage was to the extent of 25-30 per cent. The spots appeared first as transparent, changing to brown colour with dark margins. The spots later coalesced resulting in defloliation and death of seedlings (Nagaraja *et.al.*, 1980, 1992).

Causal organism : *Drechslera sorokiniana* (Sacc) Subram & Jain. (*Cochliobolus sativum* (Ito & Kurib) Drech Ex Dast. Conidia are dark olivaceous brown, fusiform, curved and broader at the centre. Conidiophores solitary and produced spores sympodically. Conidia 16.6-60.9 x 11.1-22.2 µm and the number of septa varied from 2-8. Average size of spores was 44.0 x 15.2 µm with five septa (Nagaraja *et.al.*, 1980).

3. Leaf Blight

Symptoms : The disease symptoms appeared as light brown, small circular spot on the upper surface of the leaves. The spots increased in size in later stage and coalesced forming reddish or dark brown to black patches of blight symptoms. The spots were of 1.5 cm or more in diameter. The dead tissues appeared firm and dry. Under humid conditions brown to black masses of spores appeared on the surface of lesions (Boruah *et.al.*, 1992).

Causal organism : *Glomerella cingulata* (Ston) Spauld.

Control : Leaf blight of *Dioscorea* species can be

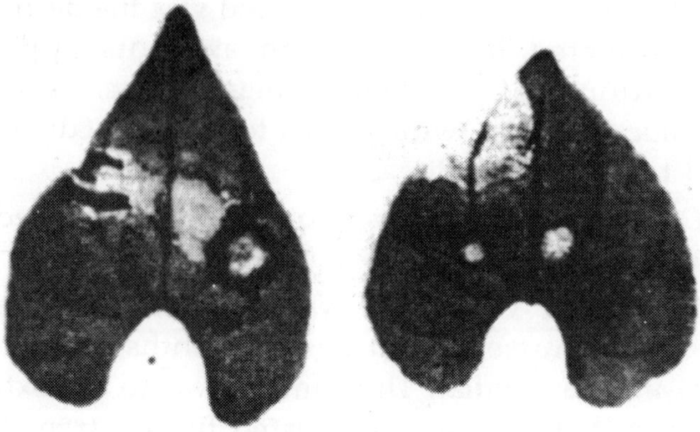

Fig. 17 : Symptoms of leaf spot of *D. composita* caused by *D. sorokiniana*

controlled by spraying with Dithane Z-78 or Copper fungicides.

4. Tuber Rot

Tuber rot of *D. floribunda* in nursery beds, fields, storage or transport is a common problem.

Symptoms : Initial symptoms of the disease was purplish brown necrosis of tissue. Rotted tissues of the tuber were soft and wet. Decay was associated with fungal infection with black masses of spores. Under humid conditions black masses on the tubers developed rapidly (Baruah *et.al.*, 1995).

Causal organism : *Aspergillus niger* van Tieghlm.

Control : The tuber rot in nursery beds, field and in storage can be prevented by dipping tuber piece in 300 μg solution of benlate or dusting with 0.3 per cent powder.

5. Dioscorea Latent Virus (DLV)

A virus with filamentous particles about 445 x 13 nm, is known to occur naturally only in *D. composita* and *D. floribunda* in Central America. The virus alone did not

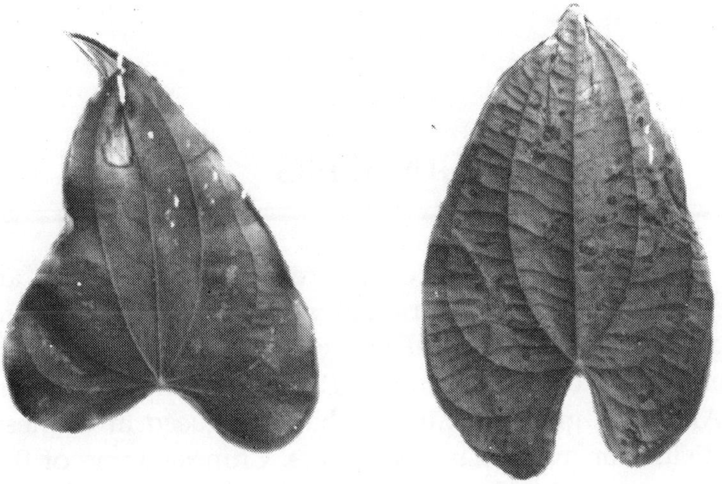

Fig. 18 : Symptoms of leaf blight of *D. floribunda* caused by (A) *G. cingulata* (B) *H. sacchari*

cause any obvious symptoms in *D. composita* and *D. floribunda*. It often occurred together with dioscorea green banding virus which induced mosaic and green banding leaf symptoms. The virus is readily transmissible by mechanical inoculations to *D. composita* and *D. floribunda*. It induced symptomsless systemic infection in *Nicotiana benthamiana* and *N. megalosiphon*. The virus is not transmitted by *Aphis gossypii* or *Myzus persicae* in either persistent or non-persistent manner. It is not transmitted through seeds. DLV has filamentous particles most of which measured 350-900 nm in purified preparations. The virus is considered a distinct, but definite potex virus (Phillips *et.al.*, 1986, Porth *et.al.*, 1987).

7
GINSENG

Ginseng has been recognized for centuries as an important plant used in oriental medicine. What is known as ginseng, is the roots of *Panax ginseng* C.A. Meyers often referred as Korean ginseng or *P. quinquefolium* L. known as American ginseng. Ginseng has been used in Chinese medicine for more than 4000 years. Chinese name of the plant was translated in the Western world as 'Man-shaped Root' or 'Man Essence' (Husain 1993). *Panax ginseng* is indigenous to Northern China and Korea. It is cultivated in China, Korea, Japan and to a limited extent in Russian countries. *Panax quinquefolium* is indigenous to Midwestern, South-east and North-Eastern USA. It is cultivated in several states of USA and Canada. Ginseng contains a number of chemical compounds. However, the activity is due to a number of saponins in the root termed as 'ginsenosides' or 'panaxosides'. In Chinese medicine ginseng is prescribed as a tonic, stimulant and aphrodisiac. The drug is considered to be an adaptogen and health tonic.

Panax ginseng is an erect, perennial herb about 60 cm high, root short, fleshy, thick, cylindrical or fusiform. *Panax quinquefolium* is an erect, 30-45 cm high, root fusiform and often branched.

Ginseng plants have been reported to be affected by a number of diseases caused by fungi and nematodes. However, only a few diseases are found to cause serious damages. Anthracnose, powdery mildew, leaf blight, damping-off caused by fungi and root-knot caused by nematodes are the major diseases of ginseng crop.

1. Anthracnose

Anthracnose is an uncommon, but potentially devastating disease of cultivated ginseng.

Symptoms : The first symptom of injury was seen when one leaflet after another turned brown, afterwards the disease spread down the petiole to the main stalk. The stalks were attacked so badly that they broke off and fell over before the upper portion wilted (Reed, 1905). Takimoto (1919) described symptoms as circular or amorphous leaf spots which turned brown then defoliated. Leaflets wilted in wet climates. Nakata and Takimoto (1922) described the symptoms as purplish brown irregular or nearly circular spots with reddish margins on leaves and stems or dark green blights on leaves. The leaf spots are sharply delineated. Concentric rings developed within leaf spots, the spots subsequently increased and crumbled, leaving holes in leaflets. Petioles and stems also developed spots and fruiting bodies.

Causal organism : Three species of *Colletotrichum* are found to cause anthracrose disease of cultivated species of ginseng (Mc Partland and Hosoya, 1998).

Colletotrichum dematium (Pers) Grove : Acervuli fusiform in outline, long axis parallel to host stem, upto 300 μm long, strongly erumpent through epidermis. Setae divergent, smooth, stiff, rarely curved, dark brown, usually 3-4 septate, 6-8.5 μm wide at the base tapering to sharpened apices, upto 3100 μm long. Conidiophores hyaline, cylindrical, occasionally septate and branched at the base. Phialoconidia hyaline, nonseptate, smooth, thin-walled, guttulate, falcate and curved, 24-27 μm long and 3-4 μm wide in the middle and tapering to pointed apices.

Nakata and Takimoto (1922) observed this disease in Korea. Miller *et.al.*, (1960) reported *C. dematium* on *P. quinquefolius* causing secondary leaf spot. Polczinski (1982) reported *C. dematium* that attached leaves and stems of ginseng plants causing spotting and blighting similar to *Alternaria* blight. The fungus was also collected in Vermont causing stem anthracnose.

Colletotrichum panacicola Uyeda & S. Takim : The original descriptions of Takimoto (1919) of *C. panacicola* is simple. Mycelia forming pseudosclerotia bearing spores and setae arise in aggregations. Setae are dark coloured at base, paler at ends, 1-3 septate, 31-144 x 2.4-8.4 µm. Spores cylindrical rounded at ends hayline, nonseptate, 17.0-22.1 x 3.4-5.1 µm. Nakata and Takimoto (1922) described the mycelia septate, hayline, 2.4-6.2 µm diameter, setae dark olive coloured, 1-3 septate, 31-144 x 2.4-8.4 µm only 2-4 septate from each acervulus, conidiophores hayline without septa, conidia cylindrical, straight or slightly curved, non septate, rounded at ends, 17.0-22.1 x 3.4-5.1 µm; chlamydospores (appressoria) formed on germination of conidia, pyriform, olive coloured, 14.0 x 8.0 µm. McPartland and Hosoya (1988) found that acervuli are erumpent, setae taper to sharpened apices, conidia are finally gattulate and apprressoria are complex with smooth entire edges.

The fungus was first collected from leaves and stems of *P. ginseng* from several locations in Korea (Chung 1974, Ohh, 1981) and subsequently from China (Li and Young 1988) Russia (Gutnikova 1963, Latysheva and Sevriuk 1981) and from Japan (Kishoi 1988). The fungus was reported to cause 47 per cent crop losses in Korea. The disease intensity increased in proportion to the age of plants and exposure to sun light and high rainfall.

Control : The disease can be controlled by spraying of Mancozeb, Polyoxin or Iprodione (Proctor *et.al.*, 1990).

McPartland (1985) isolated *Colletotrichum coccodes* (Wallroth) Hughes from Wisconsin soil previously planted ginseng. Whether *C. coccodes* actually causes ginseng disease cannot be ascertained, because no pathogenicity studies were carried out. The pathogen commonly causes root rot of solanaceous crops (McPartland and Hosoya, 1998).

2. Powdery Mildew

A powdery mildew disease was observed on American ginseng (*Panax quinquefolium*) plants in British Columbia, Canada. The disease was found where three year old plants were growing on raised beds under artificial shades.

Symptoms : The upper surface of 5 to 10 leaflets of the plants was covered with colonies of extensive white superficial mycelium. The leaves became yellow and fell prematurely. No infection of berries or stems were observed. The fungus was identified as a species of *Erysiphe*. The disease is believed to cause severe damage to seed production, root weight and winter hardiness of ginseng plants (Solberg *et.al.*, 1966).

Causal organism : Erysiphe panax Bai & Wang. The fungus produced abundant cylindrical to oblong arthroconidia 60-10 µm long and 8.0-8.5 µm in diameter. Yellow to brown speherical cleistothecia – like ascocarps were found in groups of 5 to 20 on heavily infected leaves. There were two or more asci in each ascocarp and appendages were hyphoid. The number of ascospores in each ascus is uncertain because few mature asci were seen but seven elliptical immature ascospores (approximately 22 x 13 µm) were observed in each ascus.

A powdery mildew disease was reported in China on both Asian and American ginseng. The pathogen was referred to *Erysiphe panax* Bai & Wang. However, it is not known that the species reported from the America is identical to *E. panax* (Solberg *et.al.*, 1996).

3. Leaf Blight

Symptoms : Infected leaves showed circular brown lesions on the leaf blades. The lesions coalesced resulting in blight symptoms, conidia of the pathogen are produced on the lesions. The pathogen also attacked the stem and produced linear, dark brown and velvety lesions. The stem lesions enlarged with age encircling the entire stem causing death of the plant. The flowers and seed stalks were also attacked by the pathogen (Nair, 1991). The disease is spread by the conidia of the fungus during the warm and humid weather, dew or rain is ideal to predispose the ginseng plants for infection.

Causal organism : Alternaria panax Whetzel. Mycelium composed of colourless, branched, septate hyphae 2-5 μm diam, sometimes somewhat constricted at septa. Colonies on agar usually producing a red pigment which diffuse

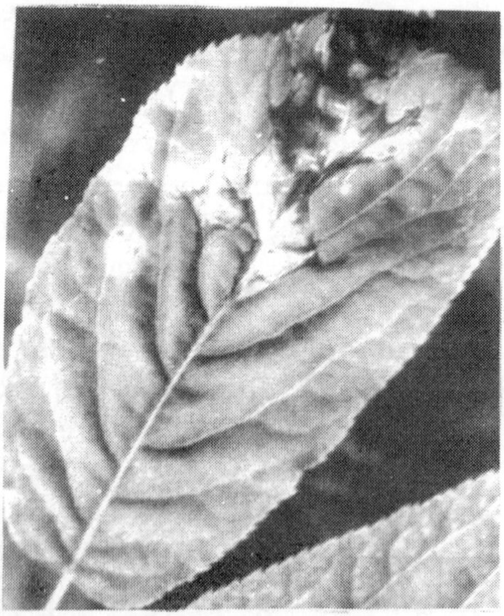

Fig. 19 : Ginseng leaf blight caused by *A. panax*

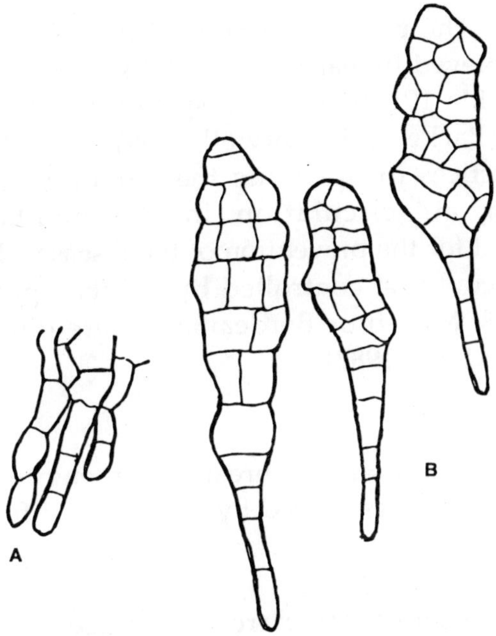

Fig. 20 : *A. panax* – (A) conidiophore (B) conidia

into the medium. Conidiophores straight or slightly geniculate, thin-walled, pale-brown, smooth, single or in fascicles, septate upto 150 (200 in culture) x 4-7 µm. Conidia solitary or in chains of 2-3, pale to dark brown, 150-160 (-190) x 12-20 µm, smooth but sometimes becoming verrucose in culture, obclavate, with 9-11 transverse and 1-2 longitudinal septa; conidial cells sometimes distending, causing the conidium to appear distorted; conidium body ± 70 µm long, with a beak which is variable in length, usually 80-90 µm long. Conidial development initiation from conidiogenous cells which are terminal at the times not, as in usual *Alternaria* by sympodial proliferation, but with the new growth repturing the apex of the old conidiogenous cell, leaving the previous conidiogenous scar at the side.

Control : The prevention and control of the disease could be achieved by early fungicidal sprays of Dithane M-45 or Kocide 101 mixed with spreader and sticker in the spring (Parke and Shotwell 1989). Use of proper cultural practices for lowering the humidity and wide spacing for air circulation in the plantation is recommended for the prevention of the disease. However, the disease could be controlled by regular spraying of Dithane Z-78, Maneb or Bordeaux mixture (Shoemaker and Konsler, 1981, 1982).

4. Root-rot

One of the most serious threats to ginseng cultivation is the root-rot diseases caused by a number of fungi.

(a) Phytophthora root-rot

The pathogen causes extreme damage during wet weather and is capable of destroying entire ginseng garden within a few weeks (Darmono *et.al.*, 1991). The disease is considered as one of the serious and destructive diseases of ginseng in USA. The spread of the fungus in the field is so fast, it is capable of attacking mature fields just ready to harvest within 2-3 weeks destroying the entire root system. Rain and cool weather are ideal for infection and disease spread.

Symptoms : The infected roots became discoloured, spongy and watery before they disintegrated. The roots show-scattered black areas which later got rotted. The infected plants showed wilt symptoms. Infected roots changed their colour and turned into soft pulp with pungent odour. The infected roots also showed disintegration.

Disease cycle and life cycle of the fungus under ginseng growing fields and disease development have been investigated (Parke and Shotwell, 1989). The pathogen can over winter in the soil in the infected underground roots. The oospores can survive in the soil for many years in the absence of the host. Environmental studies have shown that the disease development is most severe at 20-24°C. The pathogen often caused foliar infection resulting in leaf blight symptoms. The symptoms develop during rainy and cool period as dark greenish-black areas on the leaves.

Causal organism : Phytophthora cactorum (Lebert and Cohn) Schroter. Chlamydospores are usually teminal, supported by long unbranched hyphae. Intercalary chlamydospores are occasionally observed. Chlamydospores are smooth-walled, spherical and appeared to have a dull yellowish brown colour, 28-56 μm (42.2 μm). Chlamydospores are larger than oospores, 18-30 μm (26.4), oogonia, 20-36 μm (27.5) or sporangia, 29-49 x 19-37 μm (35.7 x 28.3). Chlamydospores are differentiated from sporangia by the absence of papilla, their large size and their spherical shape. The presence of a hyphal septum distinguishes the chlamydospores from frequently observed hyphal swellings in other species of *Phytopthora*. In contrast to oogonia, chlamydospores are spherical instead of pyriform, not associated with antheridia, borne terminally instead of laterally and do not contain oospores. The chlamydospore wall is composed of two layers, thin outer layer and a thicker inner layer. Oospore are surrounded by periplasm and the persistant oogonial wall (Darmono and Parke, 1990).

Phytophthora cactorum was found present in the forest soils near areas of ginseng cultivation in United States (Darmono *et.al.*, 1991). The fungus infected more than 150 plant species (Nienhaus, 1960). In general the pathogen is considered to exhibit pathogenic specialization.

Phytophthora cactorum also caused leaf blight of ginseng. The symptoms develop during rainy cool seasons. The infection caused dark-greenish-black spots on the

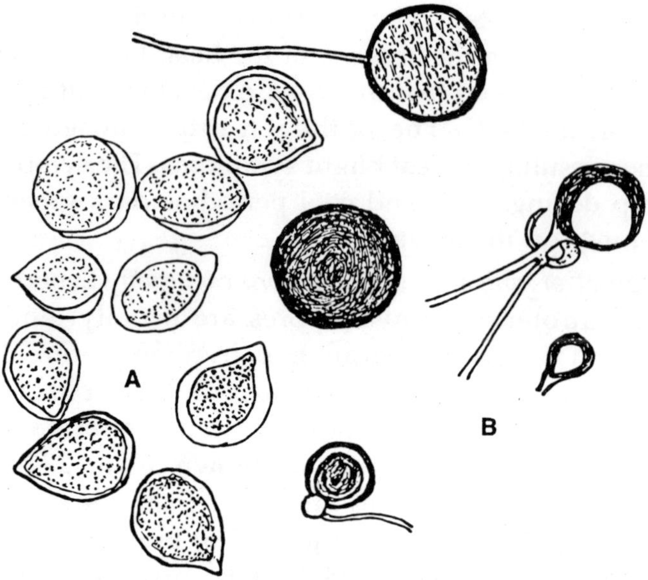

Fig. 21 : *P. cactorum* – (A) sporangia (B) oogonia and oospores

leaves. The spots later turned to brown due to the death of leaf tissues. The infection is caused during heavy rains and the zoospores get splashed to leaf surface. Infected lesions on the leaves could produce additional inoculum which resulted in the spread of the disease to other plants.

Control : Fumigation of soil with fumigants such as Verlox, Mylore, Vapam, etc. showed very effective control of root-rots caused by *P. cactorum* in large scale forest nurseries. In Japan, Korea and China, cultural practices such as deep furrows between the beds for sufficient drainage were found useful to prevent the disease. Regular spray of protectant fungicides and also the application of systemic fungicides are recommended for the control of the disease. For the control of the leaf blight, foliar spray application of systemic fungicides are recommended (Nair, 1991).

(b) Fusarium root-rot

Fusarium root-rot of ginseng was reported from Korea. Investigations were carried out in three major ginseng producing areas showed that *Fusarium* propagules were abundant in the soils of ginseng fields and in the soils of fields first planted ginseng crops (Shin *et.al.,* 1986). The number of propagules of the pathogen was 1.9 to 2.6 times higher in replanted fields when compared to first planted fields.

Causal organism : Fusarium solani (Mart) Sacc.

No reports are available on the control of *Fusarium* root-rot of ginseng. However, usual practice of fungicidal treatment of soil borne diseases would be effective to control the disease. Attempts have been made to identify sources of resistance against root-rot pathogen. Some breeding lines have recently been identified to show resistance fo *F. solani* (Cheon and Kim, 1990).

(c) Cylindrocarpon root-rot

Cylindrocarpon causes rusty orange brown lesions on the roots of ginseng. The infection often caused distortion of roots. During the early stages of disease development, the outer layers of the roots were affected and later the infection spread to deeper. The infected plants do not sprout in the next spring. They usually die as a result of etiolation and wilt.

Causal organism : Cylindrocarpon destructans (Zinssm) Scholten.

Confusion still exists as to the cause of *Cylindrocarpon* root-rot of ginseng. Another root-rot causing fungus, *Fusarium* is often found associated with *Cylindrocarpon* in this disease. The disease probably might be a complex (Shin *et.al.,* 1986, Parke and Shotwell, 1989). However, *Cylindrocarpon* sp that cause root-rot of ginseng in Japan has been considered as a new isolate of the fungus. The Japanese isolate has been designated as *Cylindrocarpon destructans* f sp. *panacis* (Matuo and Miyazaw, 1984).

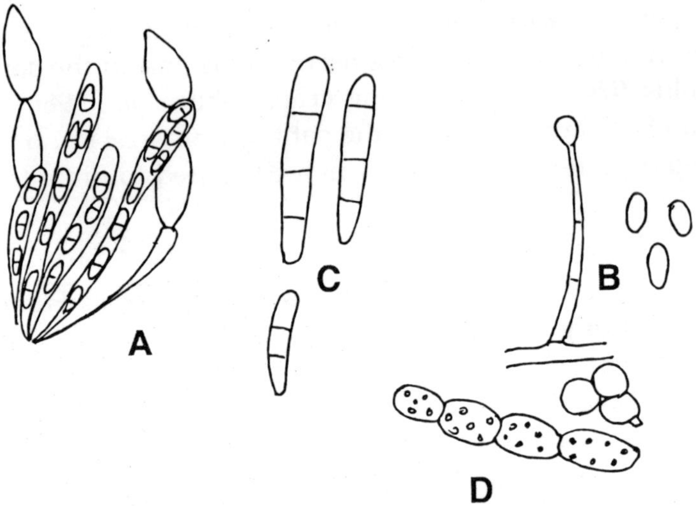

Fig. 22 : ***C. destructans*** **– (A) asci and ascospores (B) microconidia (C) macroconidia (D) chlamydospores**

5. Root-knot

The root-knot nematodes are present in various soil types. The affected plants show discolourization, stunting and wilting with roots showing characteristic nodule-like swellings called galls. The nematodes attack ginseng roots as soon as they are hatched from the eggs. The infected roots produced numerous galls. The disease is caused by *Meloidogyne* spp. Suggested control measures are selection of disease-free planting areas, sanitation of farm impliments and fumigation of soils with nematicide (Nair, 1991).

6. Damping-off

Seedling of ginseng are often infected by several fungi. Post and pre emergence damping-off are common in ginseng seedlings. Soil borne pathogens such as *Pythium* sp. *Rhizoctonia solani* and *Phytophthora* sp. are found to be associated with damping-off diseases. Soon after germination young roots are attacked by the pathogens causing discolourization and root-rot. *Rhizoctonia solani* which is present in the straw on the seed beds attacks the seedlings. Lesions are produced on the succulent stem. Use of fresh straw on the seed beds is recommended to minimize the disease incidence (Nair, 1991).

7. Black Root-rot

Ginseng is found to be affected by black root-rot disease. The disease is caused by *Sclerotinia panacis*. Infected roots showed spongy and watery with black colour. The fungus produced numerous sclerotia. The disease developed usually in spring. One of the control measures recommend is sanitation by avoiding exchange of soil or infected roots between healthy and diseased areas (Parke and Shotwell, 1989).

8
GLYCYRRHIZA

Dried rhizomes and roots of *Glycyrrhiza glabra* Linn. in known as Liquorice in commerce. The word glycyrrhiza is of Greek origin meaning sweet. Liquorice has been used in medicine more than 4000 years. The earliest record of its use in medicine dates back to 2100 B.C. Hippocrates (400 B.C.) mentioned its use as remedy for ulcers and quenching of thirst. In Greek medicine liquorice was considered as an important drug. It was used in Arab system of medicine for more than 600 years from where it was adopted to modern medicine. Liquorice is a perennial herb or undershrub. It is widely distributed in Spain, Italy, Greece, Syria, Iraq, Afghanistan, parts of Soviet Union and China. It is cultivated in a limited extent and bulk of world requirement is obtained from wild sources. The plant has recently been introduced to cultivation in Northern India. The main constituents of liquorice is a saponin-like glycoside, glycyrrhizin. Liquorice is used both in medicine and flavour. It is used in expectorants and anti-inflammatory component in cough mixtures. It is also used as laxative and treatment of peptic and duodenal ulcers. Glycyrrhetic acid obtained from liquorice is used as anti-inflammatory compound. In traditional system of medicine liquorice is used as demulcent, expectorant, antitussive, laxative and sweetener. Although liquorice and its products are used widely in medicine, the bulk of its production is used in food and flavour industries (Husain, 1993).

Glycyrrhiza glabra has been reported to be affected by several diseases. Major diseases are leaf spots and rust.

1. Leaf Spot

Symptoms : The infection produced dark brown spots on lower surface of the leaves. The spots coalesced and became dark brown lesions. The infected leaves dried and ultimately shed. The infection caused heavy defoliation (Khan and Kamul, 1982; Jain, 1987).

Causal organism : Cercospora cavarae P.& D. Sacc

Control : Fungicidal spray with Dithane Z-78 or Dithane M-45 (0.2%) is recommended for the control of the disease. Bavistin (0.1%) followed by Deltan (0.3%) is also reported to be effective to control the infection (Patel *et.al.*, 1991).

2. Leaf Blight

Leaf blight is another severe disease affecting the foliage of liquorice.

Symptoms : Initial symptoms consist of pin head size dark brown spots. The spots later developed into circular to irregular shapes of 2-3 mm size on both surfaces of leaves. The lesions were dark brown in the centre and surrounded by light brown margins. A large number of pycnidia developed on both sides of the spots. The disease was first observed in Himachal Pradesh, India (Paul and Bhardwaj, 1992).

Causal organism : Phyllosticta glycyrrhizae (Hollos) Comb. nov. Pycnida were submerged to erumpent, globose, dark and measured 54-90 µm diameter. Pycnidiospores were globose to cylindrical ovoid and measured 3-12 x 3-6 µm.

Control : Spraying of the infected plants with Cuperox or Blitox (0.2%) 3-4 times at an interval of six days after the appearance of symptoms is found to control the disease (Legha *et.al.*, 1995).

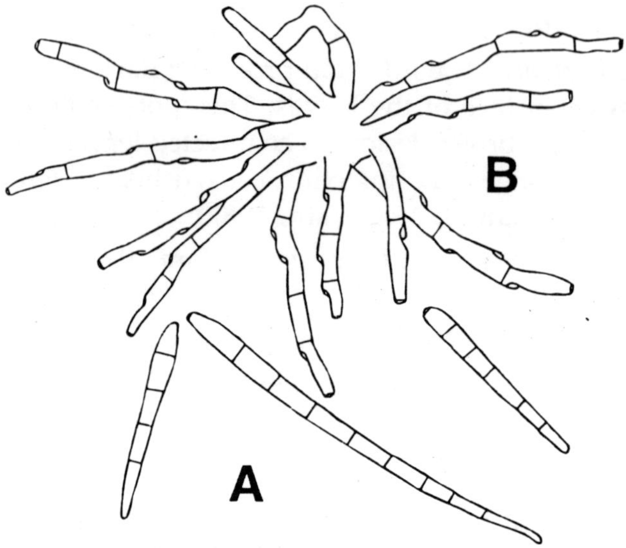

Fig. 23 : *C. cavarae* – conidia and conidiophores (A) conidia (B) conidiophores

A second leaf blight causing considerable damage to liquorice crop has been reported from Egypt.

Symptoms : Symptoms consist of light brown to black spots on the leaves and stem in the late stage of the season. The spots coalesced resulting in blight symptoms (Khadar and Abdel-Karer, 1974).

Causal organism : Alternaria alternata (Fr.) Keissler.

Control : Spraying with Cuperox or Blitox (0.2%) 3-4 times at an interval of 6-7 days is found to control the disease.

3. Rust

Symptoms : Severe systemic and locolized rust infection was reported on many wild and cultivated liquorice plants (*G. glabra*) in Southern Italy. The fungus grows systemically in the shoots, mainly in the bark and phloem and in the parts of roots nearest to the crown, mainly in the xylem where it overwinters. Besides, the typical foliar pustules, the fungus induces elongation, rosetting, defoliation, browing of the pith and formation of many buds in the crown region. From these buds infected tillers grow in spring which constitute the source of primary infection (Casulli and Ippolito, 1995).

Causal organism : Uromyces glycyrrhizae (Rab) Magn.

4. Root-rot, Collar-rot and Wilt

Symptoms : The disease started from the planting time. In case of serious infection, complete rotting of the roots was observed, eventually death and decay of whole plant occurred. Infection often spread to the stem and branches of the plants. Dark brown spots were found in the collar region. The collar portion of the infected plants occasionally girdled with the fungus.

Causal organisms : This disease is reported to be caused by a complex group of fungi which were identified

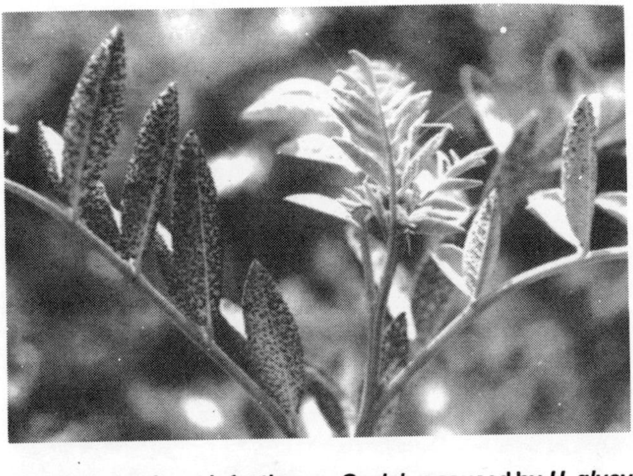

Fig. 24 : Symptoms of rust infection on *G. glabra* caused by *U. glycyrrhizae*

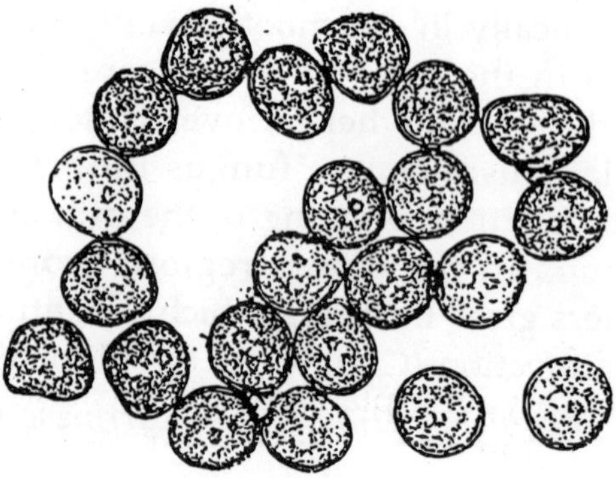

Fig. 25 : *U. glycyrrhizae* – uredospores

as *Sclerotium* spp. and *Fusarium* spp in addition to *Rhizoctonia bataticola* (Legha *et.al.*, 1995).

Control : Soil treatment with Bavistin or Benlate is recommended before planting. In case of collar-rot, removal and destruction of aerial portion above the collar region is recommended. Carbendazin (0.05%) is reported to provide control of the disease to a limited extent (Anonymous, 1984).

9
HYOSCYAMUS

Hyoscyamus species are sources of tropane alkaloids. They have been used by ancient people of Mesopotamia and Egypt more than 4000 years ago. *Hyoscyamus niger* L (Black henbane) is a native of Scandinavia, England, Mediterranean region, North America and West Asia. The plant is erect tall herb and is cultivated in USA, India and East European countries to a limited extent. *Hyosycamus muticus* L (Egyptian henbane) is indigenous to Egypt, Sudan, Syria, Afghanistan. The plant was used in Egyptian medicine more than 4000 years ago. It has been adopted to modern medicine recently. *Hyoscyamus muticus* is a perennial erect herb. *Hyoscyamus* species are raw material for the production of tropane alkaloids such as hyoscine, hyoscyamine and atropine. The flowering tops of *Hyoscyamus* species contain 0.1% to 1.5% tropane alkaloids. The therapeutic use of hyoscyamus is comparable to that of belladonna. The action of hyoscyamine is modified by the presence of comparatively larger quantity of hyoscine which produces central narcotic effects. Hyoscyamine has narcotic and mydriatic properties. It is principally employed as a sedative in conditions like asthma and whooping cough. It is also used to relieve pain. *Hyoscyamus muticus* is mainly used for the extraction of hyoscyamine which is subsequently converted to atropine sulphate (Husain, 1993).

Hyoscyamus niger and *H. muticus* are reported to be affected by a number of diseases caused by fungi, bacteria and viruses.

1. Leaf Spot

The disease was first reported on *H. niger* by Padwick and Merh (1943). Ganguly and Pandotra (1962) also found this disease prevalent in Jammu and Kashmir on *H. niger* especially in the shady localities.

Symptoms : The disease appeared as orbicular zonate, buff to woody brown spots on the leaf lamina. The spots gradually enlarged and coalesced. In young plants death of leaves due to severe spotting is common.

Causal organism : Ascochyta kashmiriana Padwick & Merh. Spores are slightly wider and measure 18.2 x 5.2 (14.8-24.6 x 4.9-7.9) µm as compared to the measurements of 19.2 x 3.8 (15.3-24.9 x 2.1-5.0) µm given by Padwick and Merh.

2. Leaf Blight

Leaf blight diseases of *H. niger* and *H. muticus* have been reported from India. The disease has a wide spread occurrence.

Symptoms : Initial symptoms in *H. niger* were tiny necrotic spots on matured leaves. The spots enlarged and coalesced which resulted in blight symptoms. The occurrence of the disease was more prevalent on older leaves. In case of *H. muticus* the initial symptoms were scattered, irregular chlorotic spots. The spots later enlarged and coalesced. Severe infection resulted in defoliation (Kumar *et.al.*, 1982, 1984).

Causal organism : Alternaria alternata (Fr.) Keissler.

3. Seedling Blight

This disease was prevalent in *H. muticus* during the early stages of growth. The disease caused extensive damage.

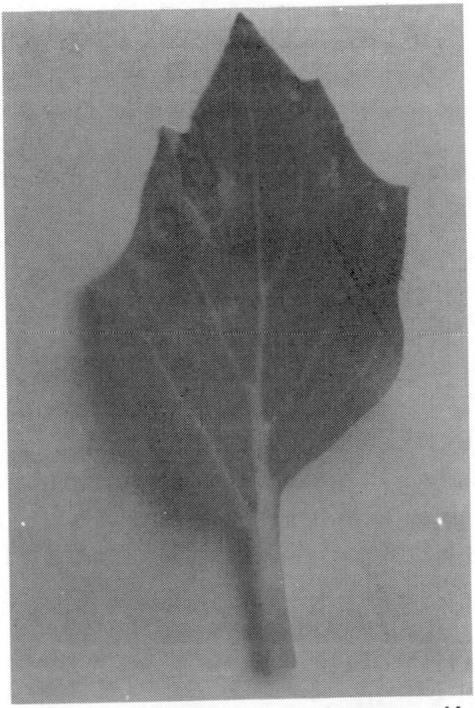

Fig. 26 : Symptoms of leaf blight of *H. muticus* caused by *A. alternata*

Symptoms : Initial symptoms appear as yellowish water soaked lesions on the hypocotyl region. The infection then moved to both stem and root regions. Infected portions became pulpy and dark brown showing soft-rot symptoms (Shukla *et.al.*, 1988).

Causal organism : *Pythium butleri* Subramaniam.

Control : Eventhough no control measures are reported, treatment of the infected seedlings with Dithane Z-78 or Dithane M-45 would be useful to check the disease to some extent.

4. Stem-rot

Both *H. muticus* and *H. niger* were severely affected by stem-rot disease. The disease incidence was severe during the months of December and January in Northern India.

Symptoms : The initial symptoms develop in the form of water soaked lesions on the above ground portion of the plants. The infection rapidly spread upwards resulting in stem-rot and decay of infected plants (Sattar *et.al.*, 1995).

Causal organism : Sclerotinia sclerotiorum (Lib.) de Bary.

5. Root-rot

This disease was found in *H. niger*. The affected plants were stunted in growth with crinkled leaves which became pale yellow. Reduction in aerial growth led to bushy appearence. Infected underground portion exhibited rotting of cortical tissue. The spread of the disease has been suggested through endoconidia (Pandey, 1995, Sastry, 1977).

Causal organism : Thielavia basicola Zopf.

6. Bacterial Blight

The bacterial blight disease of *H. muticus* was observed in India. The disease was serious and affected 50-60 per cent plants growing in the experimental plantations.

Symptoms : The disease was characterised by the appearance of water soaked lesions on the main stem. The infection gradually expanded to the branches. Infection invariably resulted in wilting and death of affected plants. Pale yellow liquid oozed from the cut ends of infected stem (Sattar *et.al.*, 1986).

Causal organism : Pseudomonas cichorii (Swingle) Stapp. Obligately aerobic, gram-negative rods, about 0.8 x 1.3 μm motile with several polar flagella, no spores produced.

Colonies on nutrient agar round, white, slightly raised, translucent, with slightly irregular margins. On

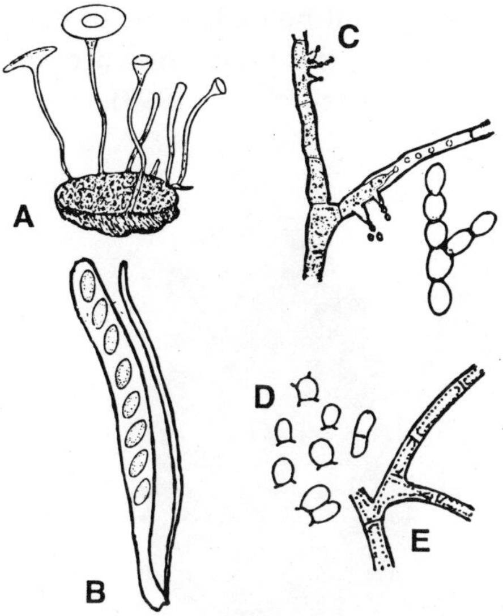

Fig. 27 : ***S. sclerotiorum*** **– (A) apothecium arising from sclerotium (B) ascus (C) microconidia (D) cells from sclerotium medulla (E) hyphae**

medium B of King fluorescent greenish pigment diffuses into the medium. On nutrient agar with 5% added sucrose colonies are not levan type (not domed and mucoid). Growth is slow in mineral medium with a single carbon source, but growth factors are not required.

7. Henbane Mosaic

Hyoscyamus species are susceptible for a number of viral diseases. *Atropa belladonna* may act as symptomless carrier of *H. niger* virus (Smith, 1945). The potato virus x and Brassica virus I have been isoalted from infected leaves of *H. niger*. Broccoli necrotic yellow virus (BNYV) and cauliflower mosaic virus (CMV) accurs together in *H. niger* (Tomlinson *et.al.*, 1927). Hamilton described the source and characteristics of three viruses found on commercially grown *H. niger*. They are named as *Hyoscyamus* virus (HYV) II, III and IV. HYV II and II are closely related and HYV IV is a different type of virus (Hamilton, 1932).

Characteristics of crystalline inclusions of henbane mosaic potyvirus showed that the inclusions are approximately 12 nm diameter (Stefanac *et.al.,* 1993).

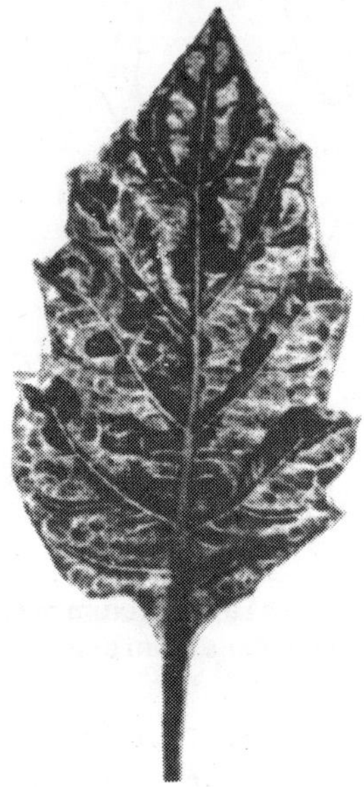

Fig. 28 : Symptoms of henbane mosaic on *H. niger*

A viral disease of *H. muticus* causing considerable damage in New Zealand was reported (Proctor, 1944). The virus was readily transmitted by mechanical means and also by peach aphid (*Myzus persicae*). The thermal death point is between 60-65°C. The control of the disease is recommended by spraying of a solution of nicotine and soft soap after a period of 8-9 weeks. Better effect was obtained by weekly spraying.

A mosaic disease of *H. niger* was first observed in India in the year 1966-67 (Sastry, 1977). Symptoms on *H. niger* consist of typical yellow mosaic mottling, vein clearing and vein banding. First vein clearing occurs which is followed by banding. The yellow colour is due to retardation of chlorophyll formation. Symptoms are typical yellow mottling. The first symptoms of the disease appeared 10-12 days after inoculation in the form of vein clearing followed by vein banding along the vein. Infected plants became slightly stunded and after several weeks exhibited yellow mosaic mottling. The electron microscopic studies revealed rods measuring 270-750 nm in length. Serological studies revealed that the virus is not related to tobacco mosaic virus (TMV) and potato virus X (PVX). However, the virus bears close resemblance in properties and host range to belladonna mosaic virus and plantago mosaic virus which are considered as strains of same virus (Chenulu *et.al*., 1968).

8. Green Mosaic

Hyoscyamus muticus was severely affected by a mosaic disease in India. The infected plants showed severe stunting and brushy appearance. The leaves were reduced in size and sometimes narrowing of the leaves was also observed. In general mosaic mottling symptoms were more pronounced in young leaves. Often the flowers became discoloured and seed setting was poor (Subha Rao and Husain, 1984). The disease was found to affect *H.niger* also (Zaim and Khan, 1988).

Based on the host range, physical properties and particle morphology the virus appeared to be identical to cucumber mosaic virus (CMV). The virus was isometric, 27 nm in diameter and was transmitted mechanically by aphid (*Myzus persica*), but not by seeds or soil.

9. Root-knot

Root-knot nematodes (*Meloidogyne* species) are the most widely distributed nematode pest. Sixty to seventy per cent *H. muticus* and *H. niger* plants in field were affected by this nematode causing chlorosis and stunting.

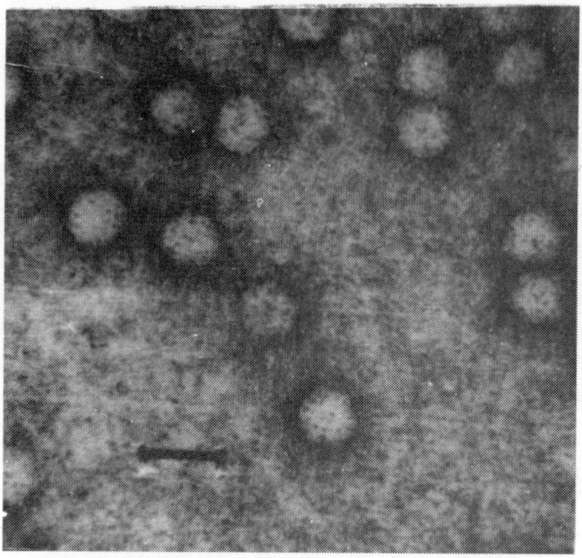

Fig. 29 : Cucumber mosaic virus – Bar = 100 nm

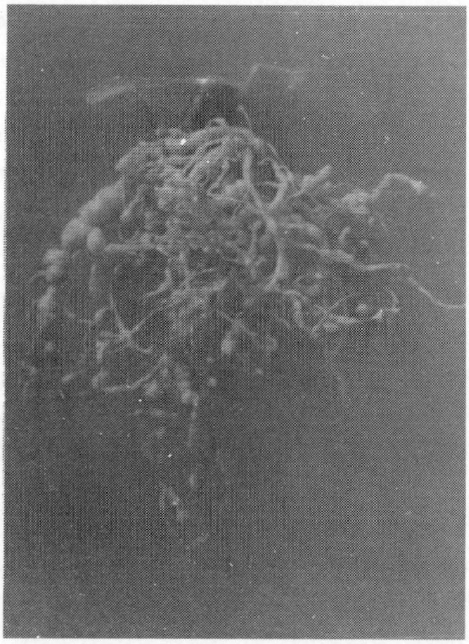

Fig. 30 : Symptoms of root-knot disease of *H. muticus* caused by *M. incognita / M. javanica*

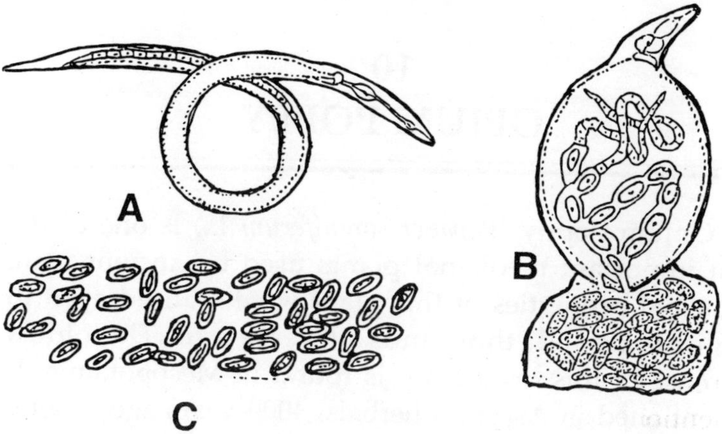

Fig. 31 : *M. javanica* (A) adult male (B) egg laying female (C) eggs

The infected plants showed root-galls of varying size on the root systems (Haseeb and Pandey, 1989).

Casual organism : Meloidogyne incognita (Kofoid & White) Chitwood and *M. javanica* (Treub) Chitwood. The former was more prevalent.

Control : Soil amendments with neem cake was found to be useful for the management of the disease. Inoculation of seedlings with the VAM fungus, *Glomus aggregatum* was found to be beneficial to reduce the multiplication and disease development (Butool and Haseeb, 1996).

10
OPIUM POPPY

Opium poppy (*Papaver somniferum* L.) is one of the most important medicinal plants used by ancient man. Medicinal properties of this plant were realised even in Neolithic period, thousands of years ago. The oldest reference of this drug plant is found in Mesopotamia. It is mentioned in Assyrian herbals, 4000 years ago. Poppy was an important medicinal plant in Egypt. The ancient Greeks were also familiar with poppy and its medicinal properties. Greeks used a decoction of the capsule as pain killer. The method of extracting the latex or opium was developed by Greeks. Greeks developed the medicinal use of opium and the Arabs developed the knowledge of its cultivation. Some believed that poppy was introduced in India by Alexander the Great in 300 B.C. However, cultivation of poppy was developed during Mughal period in the 13th century AD.

Opium poppy is believed to be native of Mediterranean region of Europe. It is an erect growing tall herb. Flowers are borne at the top of the long usually smooth stalk. Opium poppy is now cultivated in Egypt, Soviet Union, India, Turkey, Yogoslavia, Australia, the Netherlands and France. It is illegally cultivated in Pakistan, Afghanistan, Laos, Thailand and Iran. Opium latex contains more than two dozen alkaloids. To a limited extent crude opium is still used in modern medicine as well as in traditional medicine. Opium is used as narcotic, sedative, analgesic, antispasmodic and hypnotic. Principal opium alkaloids simultaneously exert both depression and exciting effects on central nervous system. The important alkaloids used in modern medicine are morphine, codeine, nascopine and papaverine. Morphine is a powerful analgesic and narcotic. It is used to relieve pain in extreme cases such as myocardial infraction and cancers. It is also used in combination with atropine for treatment of renal colic and coronary thrombosis. Codeine is used both as analgesic as well as antitussive to relieve persistant cough. Papaverine is used as smooth muscle relaxant in asthmatic, gastric intestinal spasms and coronary ailments. Nascopine is used as an antitussive in whooping cough, asthma and head-ache.

A number of phytopathogenic fungi, bacteria and viruses are known to infect opium poppy causing severe damage to the crop. Majority of the diseases are caused by fungi. Some of the diseases affecting this crop are seedling blight, leaf spot, leaf blight, downy mildew, powdery mildew, wilt, root-rot, capsule-rot, bacterial soft-rot and mosaic diseases. Among these downy mildew, powdery mildew, leaf blight and bacterial soft-rot are major diseases.

1. Seedling Blight and Damping-off

Seedling blight of opium poppy was reported to be a serious disease in Australia. Species of *Pythium* were responsible for the disease. Several pathogenic strains of the fungus were shown to play significant role in the crop stand (Angell, 1950).

Causal organism : *Pythium ultimum* Trow, *Pythium mamillatum* Meurs.

Commercial cultivation of opium poppy in Uttar Pradesh (India) were recently found to be affected by a damping-off disease. The disease occurred during emerging stage of the seedlings, mostly 2-4 weeks after sowing. The pathogen caused both pre and post-emergence damping-off (Alam, *et.al.*, 1996). The symptoms consisted of rotting of roots and collar region leading to death of seedlings.

Causal organism : Pythium dissotocum Drechsler.

Control : Treatment of seeds with Ridomil MZ-72 WP at 0.12 g/100 g seeds is reported to control the disease. Seed treatment with Captan (0.3%) or soil drenching propamocarb hydrochloride (0.3%) also gave satisfactory control of the disease. The damping-off disease of opium poppy could be effectively managed by macozeb treatment (Alam *et.al.*, 1998).

2. Leaf Spots

A leaf spot disease of opium poppy was observed in Romania and Bulgaria (Savulescu 1932, Kovachevsky 1936, Kochman 1936). The symptoms are characterised by cholortic and necrotic areas on the foliage. The infection was often accompanied by curling. Sori in the leaves formed round yellow, later grey or brownish spots.

Causual organism : Entyloma fuscum Schorter : Ustilospores globose or polygonal, hyaline, colourless, then brown, 11-17 µm thick, 2 layered, the endospores uniformly less than 1 µm thick, exospore uniform thicker and smooth. Conidia on the host on the underside of the leaves, cylindrical, curved, attenuated towards the base simple or septate, hyaline, 10-20 x 3.0 µm.

Leaf spot diseases caused by *Cercospora papaveri, C. purpurea* and *Alternaria brassicae* have also been reported from India, Pakistan and Germany (Pavgi and Upadhyay, 1964, Zaman and Khan, 1969, Grummer, 1953).

However, all the leaf spot diseases observed till now on this crop are of minor importance, though there is a distinct correlation between leaf-spot infection and morphine (Miczulska, 1967) codeine and thebaine (Felklova, 1977) contents.

3. Leaf Blights

Leaf blight disease of opium poppy was reported destructive in Bulgaria, Switzerland, Czechoslovakia, The Netherlands, Romania and Yugoslavia. Girzitska (1928), Darpouse (1945), Meffert (1949), Ballarin (1950), Milatovic (1952), Bogarada *et.al.*, (1971) and Nikitina and Vakhrusheva (1975) observed that opium poppy plantations were severely demaged by leaf blight diseases.

Symptoms : Symptoms of the disease appeared as diffused yellow spots, followed by premature drying of the infected leaves. The mycelium from infected leaves advanced to the stem, on which the pathogen produced the perithecia. The pathogen penetrated the foliar tissues and ramified through the intercullar spaces. Mraz (1960) recorded the incidence of the disease varied from 2.48 to 98.75% depending upon the locality. The infection was favoured by high temperature and heavy rainfall, particularly in July. Higher rainfall and relative humidity in June or July favoured infection (Bogarada *et.al.*, 1971). Redulescu and Perseca (1964) found that high plant density and poor nutrition favoured the infection in Romania.

The fungus attacks all parts of above and below ground parts of the plants. Seedlings are damped-off, gridling infections of the roots caused above ground collapse. Spotting is caused on leaves, stem and capsules. Primary infection was through ascospores in the spring, conidia caused secondary infections.

Causal organism : Helminthosporium papaveris Saw. (Perfect state : *Pleospora papaveraceae* (de Not.) Sacc.).

Pseudothecia immersed or superficial, single or in groups, globose to depressed globose, 300-400 x 250-

300 μm, with papillate ostiole. The wall is composed pseudoparenchymatus, isodiametric cells. Asci cylindrical bitunicate, short stalked, 4-8 spored, 100-130 x 8-12 μm. Ascospores elliptical yellow to brown, uniseriate in the ascus, 3 septate with a vertical septum usually in the two central or in one of them, constricted at the septa, 20-25 x 6-9 μm. Pseudoparaphyes filiform, hyaline, branched.

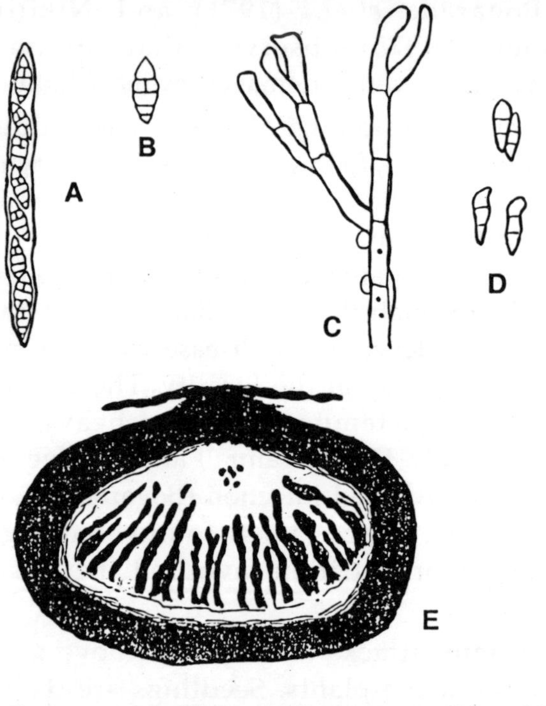

Fig. 32 : ***P. papaveracea*** **(A) ascus (B) ascosopres (C) conidiosphore (D) conidia (E) pseudothecium**

Conidial colonies effuse, black, hairy, stromata formed on stems composed of groups of a few large, dark brown cells, conidiophores variable, often in fascicles, golden brown or straw coloured, up to 600 μm long tapering towards the apex, septate, branched, conidiogenous cells polytretic, terminal and intercalary on branches, sympodial, cicatrized. Conidia solitary or in chains, cylindrical, rounded at the ends or obclavate, pale olivaceous, 3-8 septate, 17-28 (60) x 5-9 μm.

Control : Early sowing was observed to reduce infection caused by *H. papaveris* (Radulescu and Perseca, 1964; Rudny, 1976). Seed disinfection and spraying of seed beds with Bordeaux mixture or other copper fungicides also controlled the disease (Darpouse 1945, Beaumont 1953). Incorporation of lime appreciably reduced the loss. Fungicidal spraying with Systax before flowering reduced infection and increased the yield. Seed disinfection with Organol (0.5 or 1 lg/100 kg seed) significantly reduced the infection (Mraz 1963). Soil treatment with borate and manganese superphosphate (30 kg/ha) reduced the infection significantly (Misko 1963). However, spraying with Germisan (1%), and dusting with Thiram, Gramisan or Agrosan were found to be the most effective control measure of the disease (Redulescu *et.al.*, 1961, Rudny, 1976). Seed dressing with Zaprawa and Nasienna-T and spraying with Synkotox and Dithane M-45 were also effective prophylacetic measures against *H. papaveris*.

A new leaf blight disease of opium poppy was observed in an epidemic form in the poppy plantations in Uttar Pradesh (India). The disease was prevalent during the winter months. The initial symptoms consisted of small greyish brown spots scattered on the leaves. In later stages, spots enlarged and coalesced resulting in severe blighting of the leaves. Infection often resulted in yellowing of leaves. Infected peduncle became pink to brown in colour. Severe infection by the pathogen was observed both at the seedling and flowering stages (Gupta and Janardhanan, 1989).

Causal organism : *Alternaria phragmospora* Van Emden.

4. Downy Mildew

This is one of the serious and widespread diseases of opium poppy. The disease was observed epiphytotic in Argentina, Germany, Iran, Hungary, Austria and India (Fokin, 1922; Yossifovitch, 1928; Moesz, 1938; Masurat and Stephan, 1961; Kothari and Prasad, 1970). The disease was first recorded in India in 1918. The disease found favourable environment in India with the introduction of susceptible varieties, the disease rapidly became serious. Downy mildew now occurs in most regions in India (Rajasthan, Madhya Padesh and Uttar Pradesh). Downy mildew caused 20-30% loss of yield of opium latex. The secondary infection of downy mildew was found to reduce 17-22% latex yield (Thakore *et.al.*, 1983).

Symptoms : The infection spread upwards from lower leaves. The entire leaf surface was covered by downy mildew coating, composed of conidiophores and conidia of the pathogen. The stem, branches and even capsules were also attacked resulting in the premature death of the plants. The infection started from the moment the seed germinated and remained during the whole period of growth (Yossifovitch 1929). Khristov (1943) reported that the pathogen often caused abnormal development in opium poppy. The pathogen also caused hypertrophy and curvature of stem and flower stalks (Fokin, 1922).

The infection was often systemic. The leaves of infected plants remained small, chlorotic and curled downwards. Heavy sporulation occurred on entire lower surface of diseased leaves. The capsule, if formed got shrinken, wringled and dried. Severely infected plants showed extreme stunting. The infected area on the leaf first became chlorotic and then necrotic with large spots. The disease caused extensive damage to the crop cultivated in most sites.

Causal organism : Peronospora arborescens (Berk) de Bary

The mycelium ramifies between the leaf tissue and sends out short and rounded haustoria. The hyphae extend to the stomata and produce conidiophores singly or in groups. The conidiophores are stout, erect, 300-800 x 10-12 µm. They are 7-10 times dichotomously branched. Fine branches curved short and diverging nearly at right angles. Conidia are borne singly on ultimate branchlets of conidiophores. They are elliptical, oval or globose, this walled, smooth, hyaline turning brown with age, 23.1 x 19.00 µm (18.4-30x15.2-26 µm). A wide variation is observed in conidial size. Oospores, 42-48 µm, dark reddish brown with irreglar outer wall, width varying from 4 to 10 µm and with irregular ridges over the surface. In early stage each oogonium is found to possess a large round body and occasionally one or more bright yellow bodies resembling oil droplets. Average size of oogonium is 33 µm diameter.

The abundance of mycelia, conidiophores, conidia and oospores on the host suggests that *P. arborescens* and opium poppy has developed remarkable adaptability. Kothari and Prasad (1970) found that *P. arborescens* is specific. The oospores play a significant role in initiating the disease and they appear to be the source of annual recurrence of poppy downy mildew. The oospores in the soil constitute a potential source of infection. Severely diseased plants appear through out the crop period and this produces large number of conidia, which in turn become a source of infection for the new crop. In addition the disease is also transmitted by seeds.

Control : Crop rotation, wide spacing and avoidance of low lying site for growing poppy reduce incidence of downy mildew (Prochaska, 1928). Seed disinfection and spraying seed beds with 0.5% Bordeaux mixture or other copper fungicides was recommended for the control of the disease (Darpouse, 1945; Beoumont, 1953). Kothari and Verma (1967) reported that spraying with Dithane Z-78, Ferban or bisdithane gave 50% control. Spraying with Dithane M-45 (1.8 kg/ha) or 3 sprays of bisdithane (0.15%) followed by Benlate (0.15%) and crop rotation gave substantial control of the disease (Leiteritz and Rodder, 1980). Seed dressing and sprays with Ridomil controlled the disease effectively (Turkuede *et.al.*, 1982). Primary infection of downy mildew was reduced by seed and soil treatment with metalaxyl. Pandey and Nigam (1986) reported metalaxyl 25WP (0.2%) spray at 20 days interval was highly effective in controlling secondary infection. However, Ridomil treatment is the most effective method for the control of downy mildew disease of opium poppy.

Higher dozes of phosphorus application to the crop was found to decrease severity of downy mildew while nitrogen increased the disease index (Doshi and Thakore, 1995).

Alavi (1975) observed that the disease was seed transmitted. He tested five fungicides and found that 3 sprays of bisdithane (0.15%) gave the best results followed by Benlate (0.15%). Crop rotation of 4 to 5 years with one year fallow was recommended for the control of the disease. Fungicidal spray with Gramisan, Germisan or dusting with Thiram, Germisan, Gramisan or Agrosan was suggested to be useful protective measures against the disease (Rudny, 1976).

Application of Dithane Z-78 (0.4%) as a drench treatment of soil was observed to be effective for controlling the infection (Kothari and Prasad, 1970). However, Captan treatment was not recommended as this fungicide inhibited seed germination of opium poppy. A three year gap in cultivation of two consecutive crops in

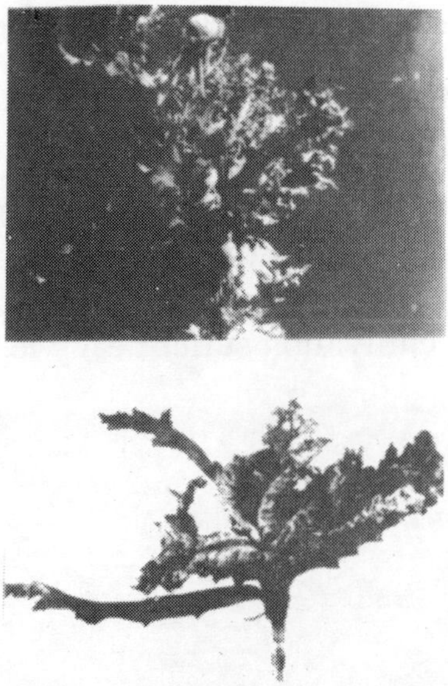

Fig. 33 : Symptoms of downy mildew disease of opium poppy caused by *P. arborescens*

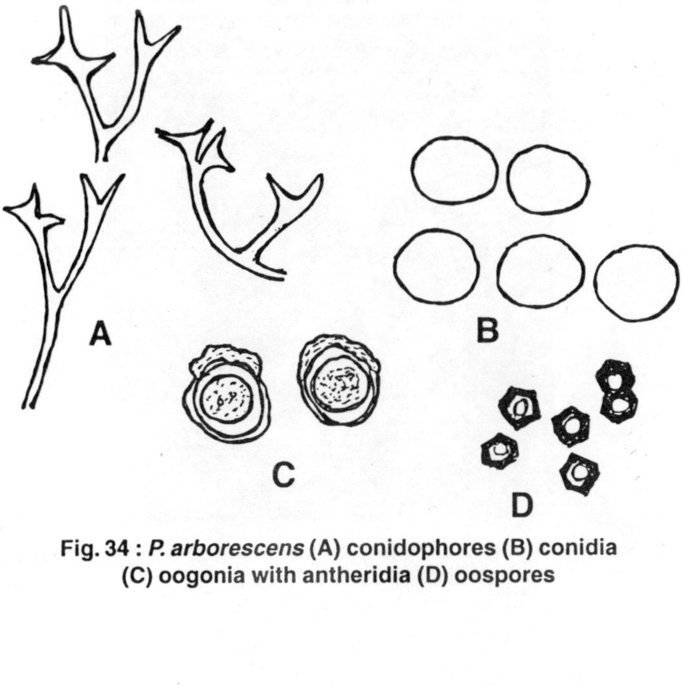

Fig. 34 : *P. arborescens* (A) conidophores (B) conidia (C) oogonia with antheridia (D) oospores

the same field and destruction of infected plants in the field is recommended as a prophylactic measure.

5. Powdery Mildew

The powdery mildew disease of opium poppy was observed in Pakistan (Zaman and Khan, 1969). The disease has been found in the severe from in many parts of India namely, Rajasthan, Madhya Pradesh and Uttar Pradesh. Poppy cultivation suffer heavy losses on account

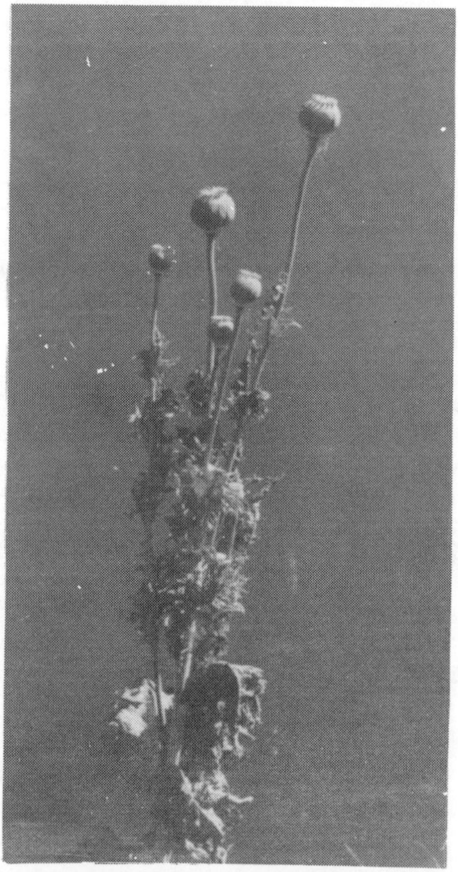

Fig. 35 : Symptoms of powdery mildew disease of opium poppy caused by *E. polygoni*

of this disease. Kothari and Prasad (1972) reported from Rajasthan that powdery mildew caused severe damage to the crop.

Symptoms : Powdery mildew disease was observed on 14-16 weeks old poppy plants. The first appearance of the disease in India is in February or early March. The base of the stem is attacked first, where it appeared as small

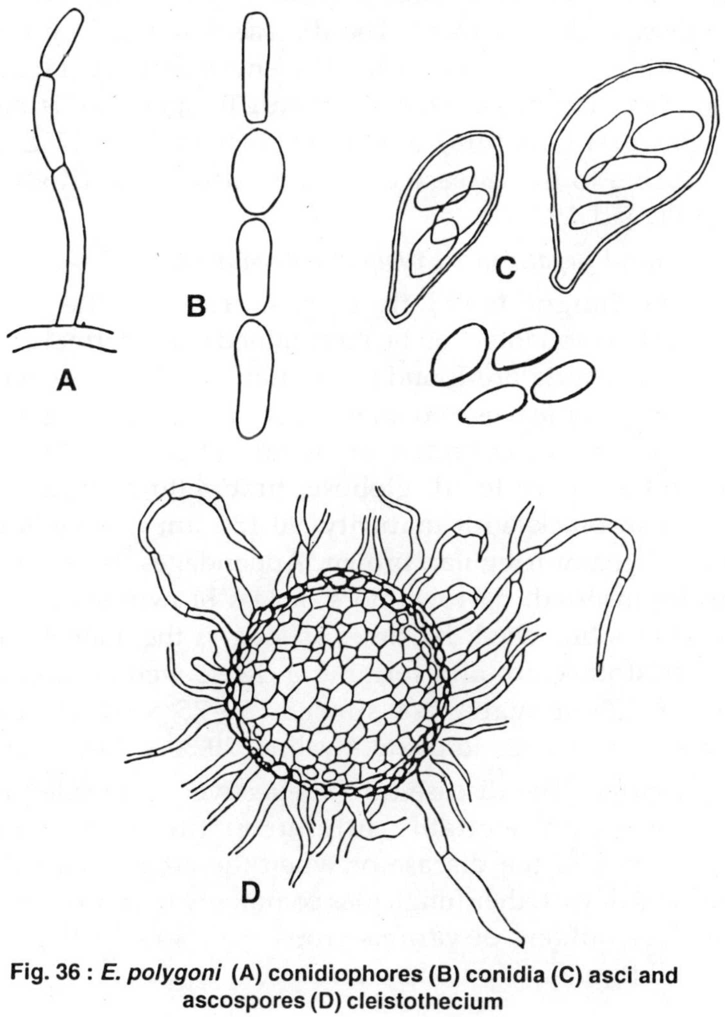

Fig. 36 : ***E. polygoni*** **(A) conidiophores (B) conidia (C) asci and ascospores (D) cleistothecium**

circular patches. Several new colonies of the pathogen continue to appear covering large part of stem. Blackening develops in the affected parts; often the stem appeared black interspersed with green patches. The mycelia spread all over the leaves. The luxurious growth of the fungus is found on the leaf surface in case of severe infection. The entire leaf surface is covered by white powdery masses of mycelium. The age of host is a strong factor influencing the disease development. The disease is never found on plants less than 80 days old. The environmental factors also affect the disease development. Temperature is one of the main factors, a temperature below 27°C is condusive to the disease development in India (Kothari and Prasad 1972).

Causal organism : Erysiphe polygoni DC.

The fungus is chiefly extramatrical on the host, penetration and infection being confined to epidermal cells where haustoria are found. Mycelium white, dense, well developed on leaves and stems. Conidia brown singly or in short chains, cylindric or ovoid, 30-45 x 10-20 μm. Cleistothecia scattered, globose, first yellow becoming brownish-black with maturity, 90-150 μm dia, cells of cleistothecium irregular, brown. Appendages, numerous, basally inserted, narrow, more or less brown, simple or sometimes branched, 1-2 times as long as the diameter of the cleistothecium and forming a dense web around it. Asci 3-12, obovate, 2-4 spored, 50-75 x 26-40 μm. Ascospores elliptic to ovate, hyaline, 20-30 x 10-12 μm.

Control : The disease can be effectively controlled by spraying 0.5% wettable sulphur at the time of the appearance of the disease or when the crop attains the age of 80 days. Other fungicides commonly used to control powdery mildew of various crops are also effective for controlling poppy powdery mildew.

Kothari and Prasad (1972) suggested one spray of Spersul (0.5%) for the control of powdery mildew caused by *E. polygoni*, while Darpouse (1945) recommended seed disinfection for the control of powdery mildew in France.

6. Capsule Infection

A large number of fungi are found to infect opium poppy capsule. Parisi Rosa (1921) observed large velvety black spots on green capsule.

Causal organisms : *Macrosporium papaveris* (Parisi Rosa 1921), *Alternaria papaveris* (Bers) Ellis (Narain, 1990), *Alternaria alternata* (Fr.) Keissler (Miczulska 1967), *Fusarium scirpi* var. *caudatum* Lam & Raw (Christoff 1934), *Dendryphion penicillatum* (Corda) Fr. (Sehgal *et.al.*, 1971)

Alternaria alternata infection significantly reduced the morphine content. Similar obsevation by Felklova (1977) indicated significant decrease in codeine and thebaine content in opium poppy capsule infected by *A. alternata*. Capsule rot caused by *Dendryphion penicillatum* is prevalent in Rajasthan (India) (Seghal *et.al.*, 1971).

Most of the capsule infection of opium poppy can be controlled by periodic spray of fungicidal formulations belonging to the group of bisdithiocarbamates. Four to six applications of 200-500 g/ha Bavistin will be a prophylatic measure for maintaining a healthy crop.

7. Wilt and Root-rots

Outbreak of wilt disease of opium poppy was observed in several parts of Spain (Navarro De Palencia, 1954). The disease occurred during the advance stage of growth causing rapid wilt and desiccation of leaves (Horompoli, 1988).

Causal organism : Fusarium oxysporum Schlecht.

Several root-rot disease of opium poppy have been reported. Severe damage to the crop was reported to be caused by root-rot diseases in Southern Europe, especially in Bulgaria. The infection originated at the stem base. Black necrotic lesions developed on the stem (Masalab 1938).

Causal organism : Sclerotinia sclerotiorum (Lib) de Bary.

Infection often originated at the stem base and was sometimes accompanied by damping-off of underground parts. Black necrotic lesions developed on the cortex of the stem (Reinmuth, 1942).

Causal organism : Pleospora calvescens (Fr.) Tul & C. Tul.

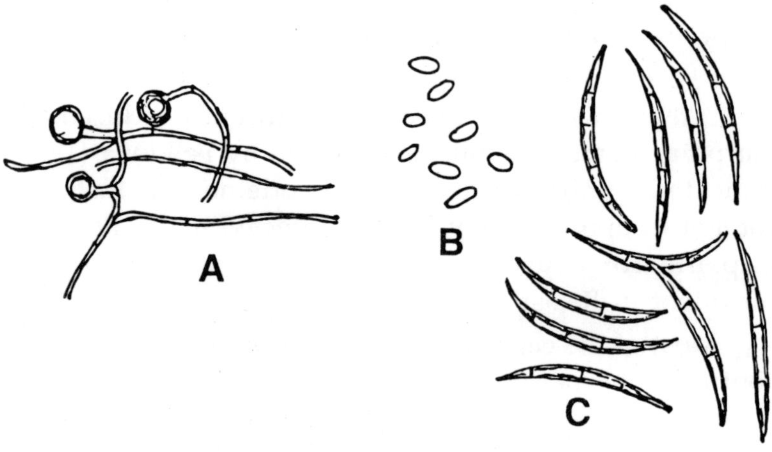

Fig. 37 : *F. oxysporum* (A) chalmydospores (B) microconidia (C) macroconidia

A root-rot disease of opium poppy was reported from Rajasthan, India. The symptoms of the disease were characterized by withering and drying of leaves, early maturity and low opium yield (Deshpande *et.al.*, 1969).

Causal organism : Macrophomina phaseoli (Tassi) Goid.

A new root-rot disease of opium poppy was found in some poppy growing areas in India. In Uttar Pradesh the disease caused extensive damage to the crop in the seedling stage. Initial symptoms were withering and drooping of plants. In later stages severe wilting observed. This resulted in death of underground parts (Gupta *et.al.*, 1986).

Causal organism : Fusarium semitectum Berk & Rav.

8. Bacterial Soft-rots

Bacterial disease of opium poppy was first recorded in Bulgaria (Christoff, 1931). The disease caused considerable damage to the crop. The symptoms were systemic in nature. The bacterium gained its entry to the host through stomata. Later it penetrated the vascular system and multiplied. The seeds from infected plants were discoloured and malformed.

Causal organism : Bacterium papaveris (Ayyar) Burgvits.

Another bacterial disease which attacked all organs of the opium poppy plant, was also found in Bulgaria (Atanosoff *et.al.*, 1932; Christoff, 1933). The bactrium caused brown to blackish-brown spots on poppy seeds and remained viable for 20 months.

Causal organism : Erwinia papaveris (Ayyar) Magrou.

The most widespread bacterial disease of opium poppy in Leningrad district (USSR) was caused by *Pseudomonas solanacearum* and E.F. Sm. *Erwinia carotovora* (Jones) Dye var. *carotovora* (Nikitiana and Vakhrusheva, 1975).

Bacterial soft-rot disease of opium poppy was prevalent in poppy growing areas in India also. Initially water soaked lesions in the collar regions were observed. The lesions spread rapidly upward and the foliage showed sign of water stress. The pith region of infected stem became soft, pulpy, often produced dirty white foul smelling exudate. Severely infected plants fell down invariably (Sattar *et.al.*, 1988).

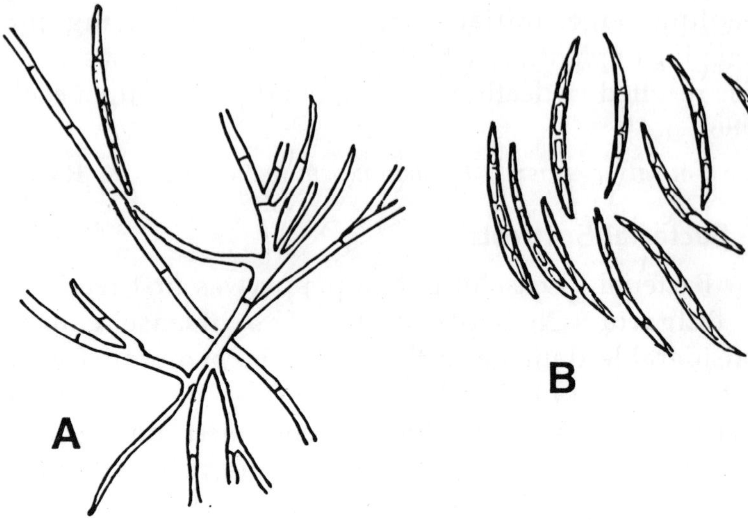

Fig. 38 : *F. semitectum* (A) hyphae (B) macroconidia

Causal organism : Erwinia carotovora var *carotovora* (Jones) Dye.

The bacterium is gram-negative, non-spore forming rod shaped, occurring singly, in pairs or occasionally short chain; motile peritrichous flagella, 0.5-0.8 x 1-3 μm size, facultative anaerobe. Colonies on nutrient agar greyish-white, smooth, round, glistening slightly raised, visible to unaided eye within 24 hr at 25-30°C. Gelatin, aesculin and casein hydrolysed, but not starch or cellulose, strongly pectotytic in pectate gels and various vegetable tissues. The bacteria are likely to be present in natural soil with decaying plant material. They are transmitted by a number of methods. They may possibly be carried by seeds also. The organism needs a wound to gain entry.

9. Cabbage Ring Spot Virus

Cabbage ring spot virus was found to infect opium poppy (Dyer, 1949). The infection rapidly became systemic (McClean and Cowin, 1952).

10. Beet Yellow Virus

Opium poppy was reported to be susceptible to beet yellow virus which was back transmitted by *Myzus persicae* to beet (Cleij, 1961).

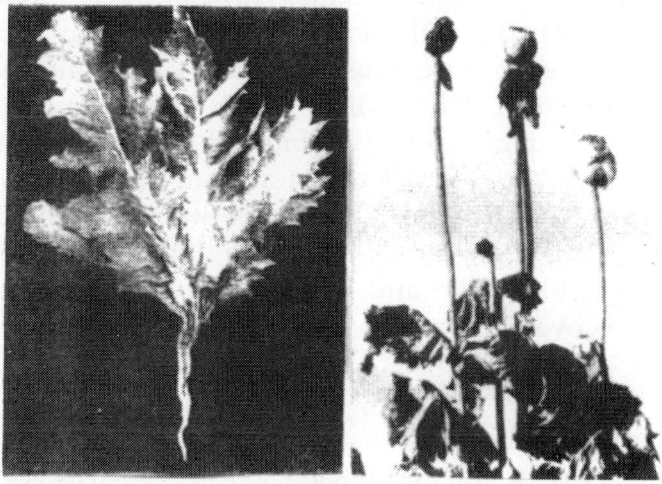

Fig. 39 : Symptoms of bacterial soft-rot of opium poppy caused by *E. carotovora* var *carotovora*

11. Bean Yellow Virus

Kovachevsky and Kovachevsky (1968) reported the occurrence of bean yellow mosaic virus on poppy in Bulgaria. Symptoms appeared as irregular chlorotic bands along the veins which spread very fast all over the interveinal areas, leaving green strips along the veins. Infected plants were stunted. The virus was transmitted mechanically by *Doralis* and *Aphis fabae* from poppy to bean and from naturally infected bean to poppy.

A virus with flexuous particle about 750 nm long, transmitted by many *Aphis* species in a non-persistant manner and also by sap inoculation. It causes diseases in various cultivated and wild legumes and also infects a number of non-legumes. The virus is common in all countries. Serological tests of the virus are difficult because it is hard to obtain sufficiently pure and concentrated virus suspensions. Strains of bean yellow mosaic virus differ serologically to various extents. However, bean yellow mosaic virus is distantly seriologically related to potato virus Y and beet mosaic virus and to many other members of potato virus Y group all of which have particles of related size and morphology. Stability of bean mosaic virus depends greatly on virus source, test plant and conditions. The thermal inactivation is usually between 55 and 60°C but may range between 50-70°C. The dilution end point is usually $10^{-3} - 10^{-4}$ and longevity *in vitro* is 1-2 but sometimes over 7 days.

12. Turnip Mosaic Virus

Turnip mosaic virus was found to infect opium poppy in Hungary (Horvath and Besada, 1975). The virus is also found to infect opium poppy in Czechoslovakia (Spak and Kubelkova, 1990). The disease is also found to occur in Turkey (Turkoghe, 1979). Infected plants showed stunting, chlorosis and distortion of the leaves, besides reduced seed and opium production. The virus was transmitted mechanically from poppy to tomato and tobacco plants.

The virus is with flexuous filamentous particles approximately 720 nm long, sap transmissible to a wide range species transmitted by many aphid species in the non-persistant manner. The virus has world wide distribution. The virus caused mottling black necrotic spots and ring spots, leaf distortion and stunting. *In vitro* properties differ between isolates. In general thermal inactivation point is below 62°C, the dilution end point in sap is between $10^{-3} - 10^{-4}$. Infectivity is retained at 20°C for 3-4 days.

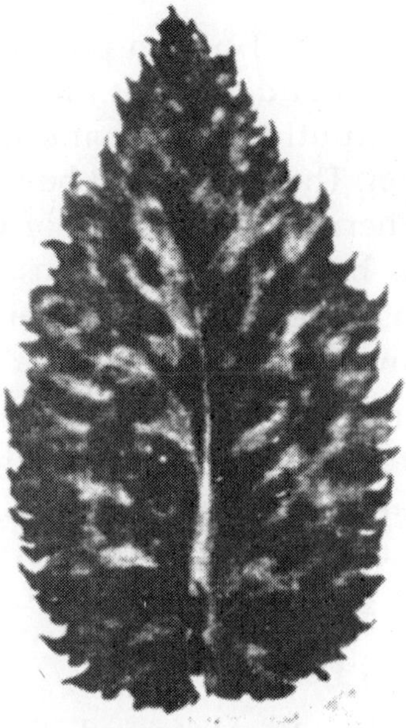

Fig. 40 : Symptoms of poppy mosaic and vein banding disease

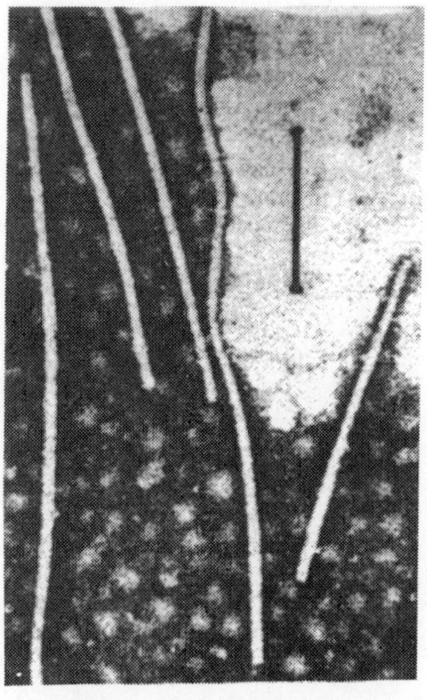

Fig. 41 : Turnip mosaic virus Bar = 200 nm

13. Poppy Mosaic

A mosaic disease of opium poppy was observed in India recently (Anand and Summanwar, 1981). The disease caused stunting, vein banding and deformed capsule formation. The virus could be transmitted readily from the sap. Thermal inactivation of the virus was 50-55°C. The virus had only limited host range. The virus also can be transmitted by aphids. This is the first viral disease of opium poppy reported from India.

A severe mosaic disease of opium poppy was observed in Uttar Pradesh (India). The virus was sap transmissible and rarely insect transmitted. Electron microscopic study showed that the virus belongs to potyvirus group (Zaim, 1989).

14. Mycoplasma Disease

Muller *et.al.,* (1974) found the occurrence of mycoplasma like organism (MLO) in the phloem tissue of infected opium poppy plants. The infection induced dwarfing and witches-broom symptoms.

11
PERIWINKLE

Tropical Periwinkle (*Catharanthus roseus.* L.) G. Don. was known for important medicinal value in folklore of a number of countries, for a long period. The medicinal value of this plant was known even in 50 B.C. (Husain, 1993). However, the importance of this plant in modern medicine was realised by an accidental discovery of the anticancer properties of its leaf alkaloids. A group of Canadian workers initiated investigations on the reported use of *C. roseus* as an antidiabetic agent. They did not find any hypoglycemic activity, instead of the extract was found to cause leukopenia in treated rats. The investigations carried out in USA also confirmed these results. Further studies by these two groups led to the isolation of two potent anticancer agents, Vincristine and Vinblastine. More than 100 alkaloids have been isolated from *C. roseus*. The leaf alkaloids such as vincristine and vinblastine are potent anticancer drugs whereas one of the root alkaloids, ajmalicine (raubasine) is used as hypotensive agent. In addition, some leaf alkaloids namely leurosidine, leurosvine and rovidine also possess anticancer activity. Vinblastine sulphate is mainly used for the treatment of Hodgkin's disease and also against lymphosarcoma, choriocarcinoma, neuroblastoma and carcinoma of breast, lungs and testis. Vincristine is used for the treatment of acute leukaemia and also for Hodgkin's disease. Periwinkle alkaloids are used in treatment of both malignant and non-malignant diseases.

Tropical periwinkle was previously known as *Vinca rosea* (L) as well as *Lochnera rosea* (L) Reich. The plant is indigenous to Madagascar, India, Israel and USA. *Catharanthus roseus* is an erect evergreen ever-blooming herb of 40-80 cm high. The stem and leaves contain a milky latex. Flowers are violet, rose, white or white with red eye. The plant can grow in a variety of climates but prefers tropical and subtropical climates. A number of diseases affecting this crop caused by fungi, viruses and mycoplasma have been reported.

1. Die-back

Symptoms : Die-back is one of the most serious diseases of *C. roseus*. Initial symptoms of the disease consist of withering of the terminal buds of young branches followed by wilting and drying of the young leaves. In later stages infection spreads downwards causing withering of entire

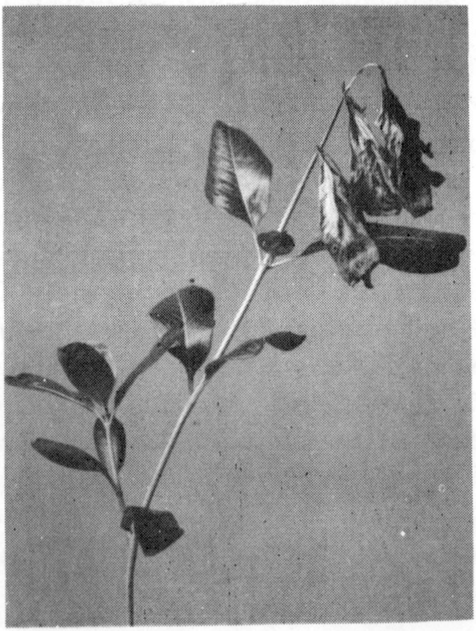

Fig. 42 : Symptoms of die-back disease of *C. roseus* caused by *C. dematium*

branch along with the leaves. In case of severe infection majority of the branches of a plant were found withered and dried (Janardhanan and Husain, 1967).

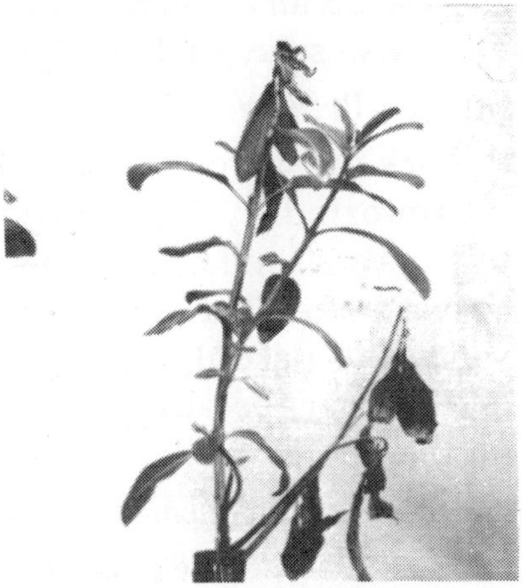

Fig. 43 : Symptoms of die-back disease of *C. roseus* caused by *P. butleri*

Causal organism : Colletotrichum dematium (Pers *ex* Fr.) Grove.

Janardhanan *et.al.*, (1977) observed another severe die-back disease of C. *roseus*. The initial symptoms of the disease consisted of the appearance of water soaked spots on young leaves. The symptoms rapidly spread to the stems through the petioles and the infected twigs invariably died. Water soaked spots were also observed on the internodal region of the terminal portion of the twig. In such cases entire upper portion of the twig died within a short period of 48 hours showing typical die-back symptoms. Nearly 80 per cent of the plants during rainy season were found to be affected by the disease.

Causal organism : Pythium butleri Subramaniam.

A third die-back of C. *roseus* was observed in different parts of West Bengal during the monsoon season

(Chakravarty, *et.al.*, 1976). The symptoms consisted of water soaked spots on the bark, 4-6 inches below the tip which gradually increased in size and encircled the young stem. Rotting and shredding of the bark resulted in wilting of the tip. The disease became severe during rainy season. The seedlings were also susceptible to the disease.

Causal organism : Pythium debaryanum Hesse.

Another die-back disease of *C. roseus* threatening the cultivation was reported by Kulkarni and Ravindra (1988). The symptoms are similar to the disease caused by *P. butleri*. The disease often became severe during rainy season. The plants are partially or completely killed depending upon their age, because younger plants were more susceptible than older ones.

Causal organism : Pythium aphanidermatum (Eds) Fitzp.

Control : Die-back disease of *C. roseus* can successfully be controlled by fungicides. Kalra *et.al.*, (1991) reported that die-back could be effectively controlled by the application of Captafol (Foltaf 80 WP). However, Bavistin 50 WP was not effective. The fungicidal application not only controlled the disease but also gave better yield. Kulkarni *et.al.*, (1992) reported that soil solarization significantly reduced mortality of plants. Kulkarni *et.al.*, (1997) found integration of host resistance with fungicide treatment would-be more effective for the control of die-back.

2. Stem-rot

Symptoms : This is a new disease of *C. roseus* recently reported. The disease was found to cause serious damage to the crops in commercial plantations. (Saini, *et.al.*, 1996). The disease appeared as pale green water soaked lesions on the stem, either below the flower head or at the collar region of the plant. Infected plants produced slimy wet rot of the cortical tissue due to which affected twigs bend downwards. The infection usually advanced both upwards and downwards resulting in slimy wet rot. In advance stage of infection slimy wet rot turned to pale, then yellowish brown and ultimately dried. Severe infection resulted in premature death of the plants.

Causal organism : Rhizopus stolonifer (Ehren) Lind.

3. Leaf-spot

Symptoms : The disease first appeared on the lower leaves as water soaked area by the side of midrib near the leaf base which gradually devloped to both the sides of the midrib extending towards the tip of the leaves. The affected leaves usually rotted, dried up and appeared black. Drying gradually proceeded towards the tip affecting the branches. Numerous small brown to black sclerotia were found on the branches. The fungus sometimes was found to infect branches also (Khatua and Maiti, 1982). The spots often developed concentric light and dark brown rings. The lesions gradually coalesced resulting in defoliation (Balasubramanian and Bhama, 1977). The disease was commonly found in rainy season.

Causal organism : Rhizoctonia solani Kuhn. (*Thanatephorus cucumeris* (Frank) Donk.)

Colonies on potato dextrose agar rapidly become brown. Aerial mycelium variable sparsely branched hyphae are frequently present. Some isolates show diurnal zonation. Sclerotia develop as crust radiating out from point of inoculation or as separate entities scattered over colony surface. Cells of hyphae at advancing edge of colony usually 5-12 μm wide and upto 250 μm long. Branches arise near distal end of cell and are constricted at point of origin and septate shortly above. Cells are multinucleate with conspicuous dolipore septa. Older mycelium shows great variation in hyphal dimensions and shorter cells owing to formation of secondary septa. The angle of branching approaches 90° and branches may arise at various points along the cell length. Some hyphae are differentiated into swollen monilioid cells often 30 µm or more in width, and similar cells derived from repeated branching of one or more hyphae from the homogeneous, plectenchymatous sclerotia. Appressoria, infection cushions and mycelium in host tissues are hyaline; the surface hyphae, which often colonise large areas beyond those penetrated and sclerotia, gradually develop a brown pigment. Hymenium a thin sheet or collar commonly on stems or leaves just above soil surface or on soil particles, discontineous, composed of barrel-shaped to subcylindrical basidia 10-25 µm long x 6-19 µm wide arranged in imperfect cymes or racemes. Sterigmata usually 4(2-7) per basidium, stout straight, 5.5-36.5 µm long, occasionally with adventitious septa. Basidiospores usually hyaline, oblong to broad ellipsoid and unilaterally flattened, prominently apiculate, smooth, thin-walled, 6-14 x 4-8 µm.

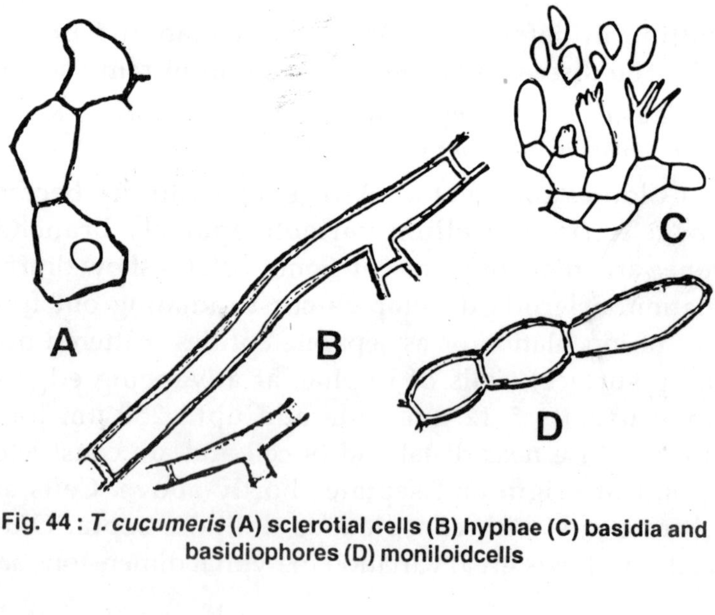

Fig. 44 : ***T. cucumeris*** **(A) sclerotial cells (B) hyphae (C) basidia and basidiophores (D) moniloidcells**

Control : *Rhizoctonia solani* is primarily considered as soil fungus. However, extensive aerial growth is possible under favourable conditions. Hence, chemical treatment of the soil and propogative materials are the most commonly used control methods. Organo-mercury compounds and pentachloronitro benzene are effective in many crops. Cultural practices such as crop rotation, shallow planting, early harvest, etc. also reduced disease incidence. Use of some microorganisms acting as antagonists against this fungus are also reported to be useful to control the disease incidence.

4. Leaf Blight

Severe leaf blight of *C. roseus* was found to occur in Lucknow (Goyal and Pathak, 1982). The severity of the disease increased in the rainy season. The symptoms of the disease appeared as small light brown spots involving almost whole of the surface of the leaf. The lesions later became necrotic with concentric rings.

Causal organism : *Alternaria alternata* (Fr.) Keissler. Mycelia olive brown in colour, hyphae branched and septate, conidiophores single or in small groups, simple or branched septate having many conidial scars. Conidia found in chains, ovoid, having 3-8 transverse septa and 2-63 x 9-18 μm in size with a short beak measuring 2.5x2.5 μm. Conidial germination was either from terminal or from intercalary cell (Goyal and Pathak, 1982).

5. Target-spot

Leaf spots first appeared as small (1-2 mm) necrotic leasions most often associated with margins of leaves of all ages. As spots enlarged, they turned brown, became round to oblong (6.45x2 cm) and assumed target like appearance. Eventually entire affected leaves turned yellow and dropped prematurally. Numerous spots were observed on leaves resulting in severe defoliation (Mc Govern, 1994).

Causal organism : *Corynespora cassiicola* (Berk & M.A. Curtis) Wei. Conidia olivaceous, obclavate to cylindrical straight or cuved, 40-190 µm long, 8-22 µm wide at the truncate base and had 4-16 pseudosepta (Mc Govern, 1994).

6. Leaf Blight

Symptoms : A leaf blight disease of *C. roseus* was reported from Cochella Valley of California. Initial symptoms were water soaked spots on the leaves. The spots enlarged and turned necrotic, resulting in typical blight symptoms (Gill *et.al.*, 1977).

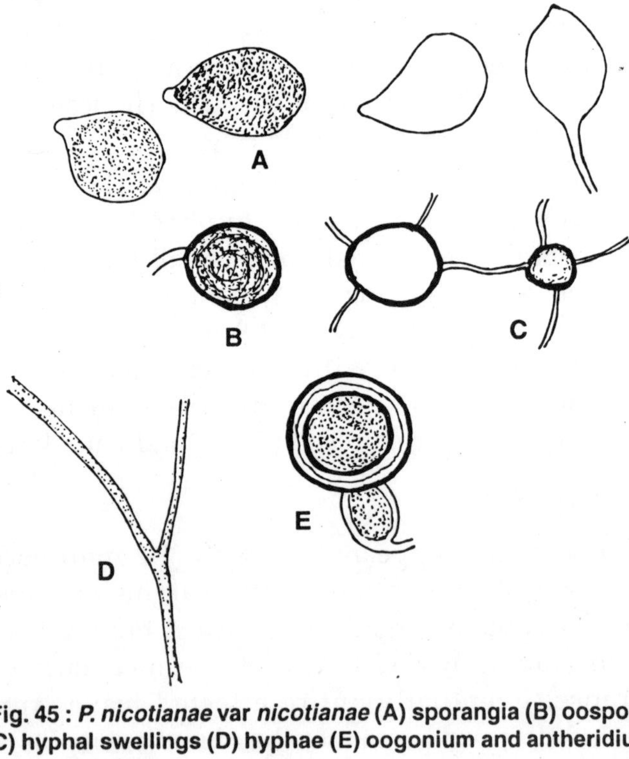

Fig. 45 : *P. nicotianae* var *nicotianae* (A) sporangia (B) oospore (C) hyphal swellings (D) hyphae (E) oogonium and antheridium

Causal organism : Phytophthora nicotianae Breda de Haan. Hyphae fairly uniform with frequent hyphal swellings upto 5 µm diam. On sporangiophores, spherical, oval or angular swellings of all sizes up to 20 µm are found. As soon as the swellings develop, 4-5 hyphae may grow out from various points. Chlamydospores frequent, formed early on the new mycelium, 20-40 µm diam, wall 1.5 µm thick, not usually turning brown. Sporangiophores thin (2 µm), closely or sparsely branched, the branches usually arising from a hyphal swelling; sporangia terminal or intercalary, broadly turbinate, the basal part nearly spherical and the apical narrowed or prolonged into a beak, 45 x 36 µm, often upto 60-70 µm long, not usually deciduous; papilla conspicuous, often two present. Oogonia formed promptly in culture by some isolates, mostly 28-30 (-32 µm) diam., wall becoming sligntly thicker with age and acquiring a golden brown accretion. Antheridia always amphigynous, but the oogonial stalk is sometimes quite eccentric so that the antheridium appears to be not amphigynous at first sight, 10-16 x 10 µm, rounded rather than angular. Oospore not filling the oogonium, 24-26 µm diam., wall 1.5-2(-3) µm thick, usually colourless or faintly yellow.

7. Foot-rot

Symptoms : This disease was observed in West Bengal (Chakravarty *et.al.*, 1976). The first symptom of the disease is yellowing and drying of the leaf tips. Young plants wilt and collapsed rapidly. The bark at the collar region is found to be rotted and white mycelial growth is found on the infected area.

Causal organism : Sclerotium rolfsii Sacc. (*Corticium rolfsii* Curzi).

8. Root and Collar-rot

Symptoms : Initial symptoms of the disease was the appearance of chlorosis on the plants. The plants later wilted gradually. The wilted plants later collapsed. The wilted plants when uprooted, severe rotting on the root and collar regions was observed. The tissues of cortical regions were severely affected by disintegration (Ravindra, 1986).

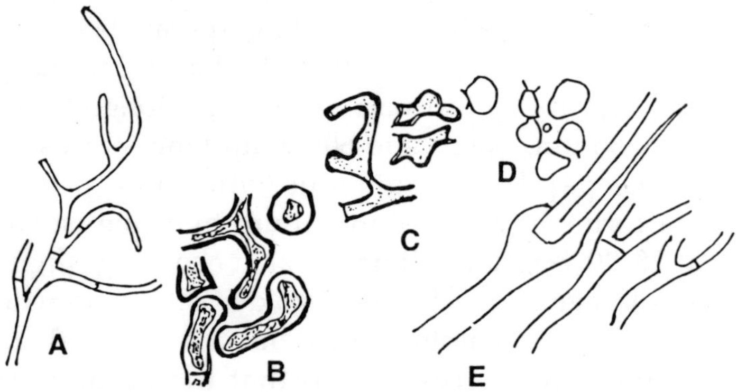

Fig. 46 : *C. rolfsii* (A) tertiary hyphae (B) cells from sclerotia medulla (C) cells from sclerotia cortex (D) cells from sclerotia rind (E) primary and secondary hyphae

Causal organism : Pythium aphanidermatum (Eds.) Fitz. Mycelium white, well developed and wooly. Hyphae upto 7.5 µm diam. Zoosporangia produced only in liquid culture, often smaller and less profusely branched than those of *P. butleri*, swellings sometimes only forming bud-like outgrowth from the main sporangial element; encysted zoospores 9 µm diam. Oogonia usually abundant in culture and in the host, terminal on lateral hyphae, 19-29 µm, wall smooth. Antheridium terminal or intercalary, barrel-shaped or broadly clavate, 9-11 x 10-14 µm, more usually produced adjacent to the oogonium. Oospore very loose in the oogonium smooth walled, 2 µm thick with an average size of 17.5 µm.

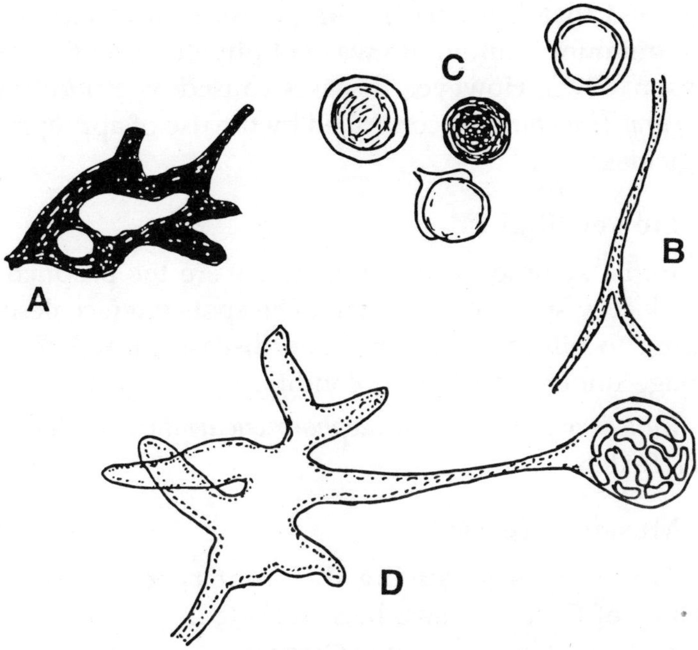

Fig. 47 : *P. aphanidermatum* (A) sporagium (B) hyphae (C) oospore (D) oogonium and antheridium

Control : Appreciable good control of the disease could be achieved by the application of fungicides. However, introduction of disease resistant cultivars would be useful. Tetraploid lines were reported to show certain amount of resistence to the disease (Kulkarni and Ravindra, 1988). A combination of resistant varieties and use of appropriate fungicides would be the most effective method for the control of the disease.

9. Damping-off

Pre-emergence damping-off of *C. roseus* has been reported to cause serious damage to the seedlings. This was reported to be caused by *Phytophthora parasitica* Dastur. Attempt was made to control the disease by aluminium sulphate drenching in the soil. The finding suggested that *P. nicotianae* var. *parasitica* was supressed by aluminium. Aluminium was not phytotoxic to *C. roseus* (Benson, 1995). However, diseases caused by *P. nicotianae* var. *parasitica* could be controlled by the use of appropriate fungicides.

10. Flower Blight

Initial symptoms of the disease were the production of dark grey spots on the petals. The spots often coalesced leading to blight symptoms. The disease caused severe damage under high humid conditions (Holcomb, 1998).

Causal organism : Choanephora cucurbitarum (Berk. & Rav) Taxter.

11. Mosaic Diseases

Three viruses causing different types of mosaic diseases of *C. roseus* have been reported.

Joshi and Raychaudhari (1964) reported a mosaic disease of *C. roseus*. The disease was characterized by circular to irregular greenish yellow to green patches and leaf malformation. The virus was transmitted by sap inoculation. The virus was designated as Periwinkle mosaic. The virus had an incubation period of 60-70 days in *C. roseus* and was not transmissable by insects. The virus produced greenish yellow spots followed by yellow streaks 8-10 days after inoculation.

Zaidi *et.al.*, (1978) reported a mosaic disease of *C. roseus*. The symptoms consisted of yellow green mosaic followed by crinkling of the leaves and general stunting of the plants. The virus was transmitted by sap as well as by insect vector. In addition to sunting mosaic symptoms were also observed. The virus differed in its properties from periwinkle mosaic and thus, it was designated as Periwinkle chlorotic stunt virus.

Verma and Dwivedi (1991) reported another mosaic disease of *C. roseus*. the virus caused severe mottling, blistering and distortion of leaves. Infected plants showed stunting, mosaic mottling and distortion in the foliage and flowers. Dark and light green areas were distinctly seen on the leaf lamina. The leaf lamina became very distorted, margins showed slight upward rolling and leaf size was considerably reduced. Flowers produced on the infected plants were smaller and distorted. Petals were narrow, reduced, twisted and closely apperessed. The infected plants showed great reduction in vegetative and reproductive growth. The virus was easily transmitted by sap and insects to a large number of plants. The virus was suggested to belong to Cucumovirus group. Plant indicators, electronmicroscopic and immunodiagnostic studies showed that cucumber mosaic cucumo virus as causal agent of mosaic disease of periwinkle (Giorgadze, 1989).

Causal organism : The causal organism was identified as Cucumber mosaic virus. The virus is a RNA containing virus with isometric paticles about 30 nm in diameter. It has a wide host range, is transmitted by many species of aphids in a non-perisistent manner and is readily transmissible by inoculation of sap. The virus is widespread and common in temperate regions. The virus is poorly immunogenic. Molecular weight of the virus was estimated 5.8-6.7 x 10^6 daltons.

12. Tomato Spotted Wilt Virus

Periwinkle (*C. roseus*) with symptoms of a virus infection were observed in Sicily, Italy in the spring of 1992. The symptoms included leaf necrosis of the blade and margin. The virus was identified as Tomato spotted wilt virus (TSWV) on the basis of transmission studies, serological tests and electronmicroscopic studies (Davino *et.al.*, 1993).

13. Phyllody

Symptoms : The occurrence of phyllody or little leaf disease of *C. roseus* has been reported by several workers from India (Chakravarty *et.al.*, 1976, Kar *et.al.*, 1982, Subba-Rao *et.al.*, 1983, Sharma *et.al.*, 1993). The disease has also been reported from a number of other countries (Grimaldi and Grasso, 1988; Dale, 1987). Typical symptoms of the disease were reduction in the size of leaves, shortening of internodes, extensive branching and stunting with greening of flowers. When the disease intensified the plants turned vegetative with complete loss of flowering and fruiting. The diseased plants often looked like small bushes with stunted growth. Excessive branching was observed the leaves turned chlorotic with pointed tips. There is a complete transformation of the appearance of the diseased plants beyond recognition from the normal plant. The disease caused considerable reduction in the alkaloid content of the plant.

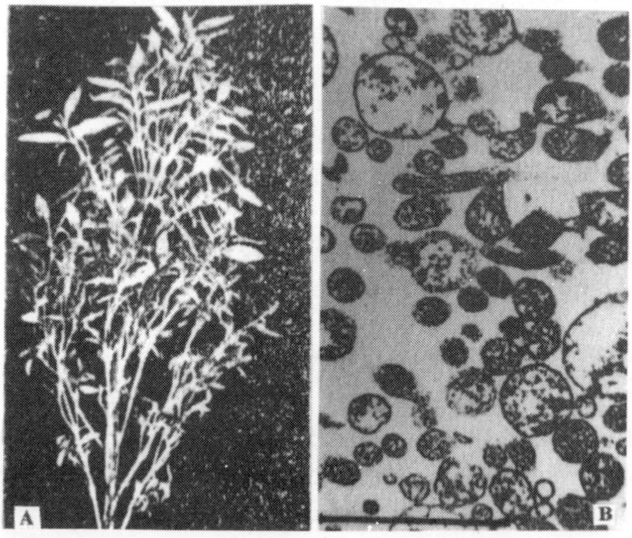

Fig. 48 : (A) *C. roseus* showing phyllody disease symptoms (B) Mycoplasma like organism in the sieve plates of infected plants

Causal organism : The causal organism was identified as mycoplasma or mycoplasma like organism (MLO). Electronmicroscopic examination of leaf tissue sections of infected plants revealed the presence of numerous pleomorphic bodies in the sieve tube cells of phloem elements. The bodies were of different sizes, most often circular and rarely oval. The bodies were bound by a unit membrane. Some bodies were found to undergo binary fission. Such bodies were not detected in other cells except in pholem.

The organism was not mechanically transmissible, but could be transmitted through grafts. Dabek (1982) reported the transmission of the disease by leaf hoppers to periwinkle.

Control : Tetracycline treatment proved highly successful in limiting the disease symptoms (Kar *et.al.*, 1983). Treatment with oxytetracycline at 500 μg caused remission of the symptoms. The treatment resulted in amelioration of the disease symptoms. Treated plants were found to produce normal leaves and flowers. Tetracycline and gibberellic acid therapy was more effective (Kar *et.al.*, 1983, Shepardson and Mc Green, 1979).

12
PLANTAGO

Ripe seeds of *Plantago psyllium* Linn. is known in commerce as Spanish or French psyllium and that of *Plantago ovata* Forsk. is referred as Indian psyllium. *Plantago psyllium* is cultivated in France and Spain for European market. Most of the world supply of psyllium seeds comes from *Plantago ovata*. *Plantago ovata* is a native of Mediterranian region especially Southern Europe, North Africa and West Pakistan. The plant is commercially cultivated in Gujarat and to a limited extent in Haryana and Rajasthan provinces of India. Psyllium has been used in traditional medicine in Middle East and in India for several hundred years. *Plantago ovata* is an annual herb with narrow linear rosette like leaves. The husk of the seeds contains a colloidal mucilage or polysaccharide mainly consisting of xylose, arabinose, galacturonic acid with rhamnose and galactose. Two polysaccharide fractions have been isoalted from the mucilage. The first fraction is soluble in cold and the second in hot water. The mucilage is thirty percent of the weight of the whole seed. Infusion or decoction of the seeds is used to control chronic constipation. It is also used to control diarrhoea and dysentry. The mucilage acts as a smoothing lubricant, absorbs toxins and relieves intestinal irritation. The psyllium seed mucilage is the main constituent of a number of laxative preparations available in the market (Husain, 1993). *Plantago ovata* under commercial cultivation has been reported to suffer from a number of diseases caused by fungi and viruses.

1. Downy Mildew

Downy mildew is the major and serious disease of *P. ovata*. It causes enormous quantitative and qualitative loss and often becomes a limiting factor in the successful cultivation of the crop (Desai and Desai, 1969). Usually the disease appears at the time of spike initiation.

Symptoms : Initial symptoms consist of small pale yellow patches on the leaves which progressively spread, completely destroying the leaves. The chlorotic areas develop in the upper surface of the leaves and ash white frost like mycelial growth develops on the lower surface of the leaves. Subsequently, infected leaves become chlorotic and brownish in colour, followed by curling, crinkling and drying of plants (Desai and Desai, 1969). Occasionally, chlorotic streaks, extending along with the midrib of leaves are observed. In such cases profuse downy gorwth is observed on the lower surface of the leaves. Ultimately, the whole leaf turns necrotic and in severe cases the entire plants appeared blighted. The abundant oospore formation caused thickening of affected leaves (Kapoor and Chowdhary, 1976).

Causal organism : The disease is reported to be caused by two pathogens (1) *Peronospora alta* Fuckel (Kapoor and Chowdhary, 1976) (2) *Peronospora plantaginis* Underwood (Desai and Desai, 1969).

Peronospora alta, mycelium intercellular, haustoria hyphal and infrequent sporangiosphores measuring 290-450 x 8.0 µm; branching obscurely dichotomus 4-5 times, branch slender, tapering and curved at an angle usually less than 90°. Oospores rarely found (Kapoor and Chowdhary, 1976).

Peronospora plantaginis, hyphae intercellular with average breadth of 9.5 µm. Sporangiophores appear slender and tree like with an erect trunk, grey to pale yellow violet in colour emerging singly or in clusters from stomata on the lower surface and were dichotomously branched. The sporangia are sub-hyaline, broadly elliptical to subglobose and measuring an average of 35 x 21 µm (Patel 1984). Sporangia upon germination produced germ tubes and penetrated through stomata. Sporangia and sporangiophores emerged through stomatal opening before the death of the tissues. Zoospore formation was never observed (Patel, 1984). Under field conditions germination of the sporangia is favoured by temperature around 20°C and relatively humidity 82 per cent.

Control : It is difficult to keep the disease under control once it has affected the crop extensively. The disease is seed as well as as soil borne. Studies have shown that high seed rate increased disease severity (Pandey 1995). Studies were also carried out to locate source of genetic resistance in the germplasm. No significant source of resistance could be identified (Desai and Desai, 1969). Soaking of the seeds in aureofungin (0.75%) solution coupled with two spraying of aureofungin at 15 g/ha controlled the disease effectively. The first spray was given immediately after the appearance of the disease and was repeated twice and at intervals of 8-10 days (Desai and Desai, 1969). Seed treatment with metalaxyl (5 g/kg seed) coupled with three sprayings of captafol (0.2%) or metalaxyl (0.05%) effectively controlled the disease (Patel 1984). The spraying was done first after the appearance of the disease and repeated at 10 days intervals. Fungicidal sprays with Bordeaux mixture, copper oxycholoride, Dithane M-45 or Dithane Z-78 would be useful prophylatic measure for the control of the disease.

2. Damping-off

Plantago ovata suffers from both pre-emergence and post-emergence damping-off. Older plants are less susceptible than the young seedlings (Chastager *et.al.*, 1979). In pre-emergence damping-off young seedlings wither they reach the surface of the soil. While in case of post-emergence damping-off the plantlets are affected first. Initial infection appeared as darkened, water-soaked spot on collar region of the seedlings. The infection extends rapidily leading to the death of seedlings. The disease normally occurred at high temperature and humidity at the time of sowing (Anon. 1985).

Causal organism : Damping-off of *Plantago* has been reported to be caused by a number of pathogens (1) *Pythium ultimum* Trow. (Chastagner *et.al.*, 1979), (2) *Rhizoctonia solani* Kuh. (Anon, 1980) (3) *Fusarium oxysporum* (Schl) Syn & Hans (Russell, 1975).

Control : Seed treatment with metalaxyl or fenaminosulf (5 g/kg) protected the seedlings to a great extent (Chastagner *et.al.*, 1979). However, seed treatment with fenaminosulf was some what phytotoxic.

3. Wilt

The disease was found either as damping-off or as late season wilting when the plants started to produce seeds (Russell, 1975).

Symptoms : Initial symptoms consist of change in colour of outer leaves from green to silver. Wilting symptoms onset rapidily. The leaves became postrate. Discolourization occurs on the tap root which is accompanied by accumulation of large amount of hyphae in the xylem vessels. Vascular discolourization and cortical root-rot were also observed (Russell, 1975).

Causal organism : A number of pathogens have been reported to be responsible for the disease (1) *Pythium ultimum* Trow. (Chastagner *et.al.*, 1979) (2) *Fusarium oxysporum* (Schl) Syn & Hans (Russell, 1975). (3) *Fusarium solani* Ell & Mart (Mehta and Madan 1985).

Control : Seed treatment with a systemic fungicide, such as bavistin or benlate (2.5 g/kg) has been reported to protect the seedlings for a month (Russell, 1975).

4. Powdery Mildew

The disease is of minor importance. The disease appeared at the time of flowering (Shankhela *et.al.*, 1985). Small white or greyish spots appeared on the leaves which gradually enlarged and eventually covered the entire plant surface with white powdery mass (Shankhela *et.al.*, 1985).

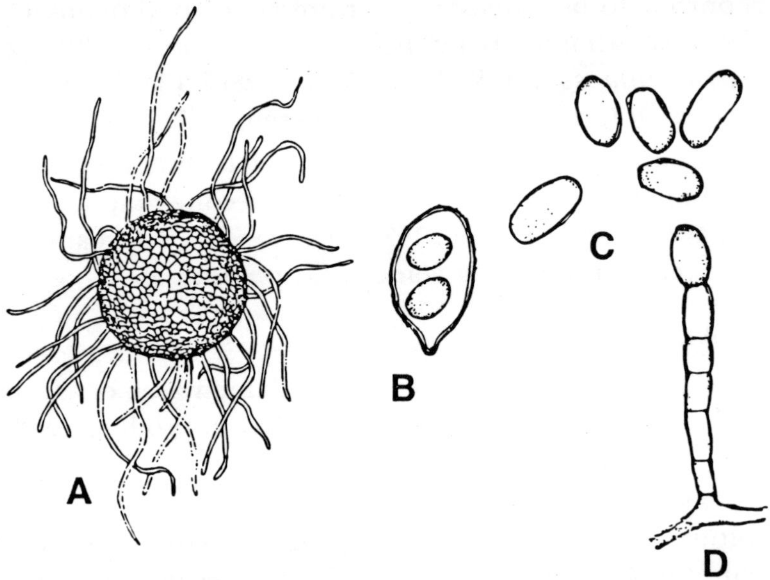

Fig. 49 : *E. cichoracearum* (A) cleistothecium (B) ascus (C) conidia (D) conidiophore

Causal organism : Erysiphe cichoracearum D. C. (Kumawat, 1979).

Control : The disease can be controlled by spraying Karathane W.D. (0.2%) or wettable sulphur compounds immediately after the appearance of the disease (Shankhela, *et.al.*, 1985).

5. Leaf Blight

The disease was reported in experimental plantations of *P. ovata*.

Symptoms : Symptoms consisted of dull-green yellowish colour on the leaf tip. The older and matured leaves were more severely affected. More than fifty per cent leaf area showed irregular necrotic spots which enlarged rapidly. In the advance stage, the leaves blackened due to blight symptoms. This was followed by death and drying of the leaves. Severe infection often caused shrivelling and blackening of seeds (Patel *et.al.*, 1984).

Causal organism : Alternaria alternata (Fr.) Keissler.

6. Viral Diseases

Eight viruses were observed to infect *Plantago*. Two of them were identified as previously described viruses : Ribgrass Mosaic Virus and Plantain Virus A. However, 6 viruses are believed to be new records. They are tentatively classified as a Potex Virus, a Caulimo Virus, a Poty Virus, a Carla Virus and two isometric viruses with properties similar to the Tobacco Necrosis Virus group and Tombus viruses (Hammond, 1981). The large number of virus types known to infect *Plantago* species indicate that the plants have a broad range of susceptibility to plant viruses and may act as a reservoir of viruses which are able to infect other crops.

13
PODOPHYLLUM

The drug Podophyllum is obtained from rhizomes and roots of *Podophyllum peltatum* L. or *P. emodi* Wall (Syn. *Podophyllym hexandrum* Royle). The durg has been used by American Indians as emetic, purgative, etc. *Podophyllum peltatum* is a herb with perennial creeping, fibrous branched rhizomes. *Podophyllum emodi* is glabrous, 15-20 cm tall more or less succulent, perennial herb with a creeping knotty rhizome bearing thick fibrous roots. The active constituents of the plants are present in the rhizomes in the forms of resin called podophyllin or podophyllotoxin which are the anticancer principles. Podophyllotoxins are used by the pharmaceutical industry for structural modifications to produce anticancer drugs, tenoposide and etoposide being marketed by Sandoz. Etoposide has been found useful in treatment of lung cancer, testicular cancer, lymphoma and leukaemia. Tenoposide has been mainly used to treat acute lymphatic leukaemia, neroblastoma and brain tumor in children (Husain, 1993). *Podophyllum* is reported to be affected by only a few diseases.

1. Rust

Mayapple (*Podophyllum peltatum*) is attacked by a non-specific rust fungus. The pathogen is potentially damaging to its host (Sohn and Plicansky, 1977). Host infection occurs via contact with spore-contaminated soil during shoot emergence in early spring (Whetzel *et.al.*, 1925).

Symptoms : Orange lesions (aecia) develop on leaves within two weeks after infection. Aeciospores shed and immediately reinfect leaves, causing scattered black lesions (telia) from which over wintering teliospores develop. The first generation of the pathogen appears to be most-harmful, since plants are damaged early in their seasonal growth cycle. Heavy aecial infection is associated with a significantly reduced plant growth (Parker, 1988). Disease impact appears to be much less during the second pathogen generation, since telial development occurs in late spring, just prior to normal leaf senescence.

Causal organism : *Puccinia podophylli* Schw.

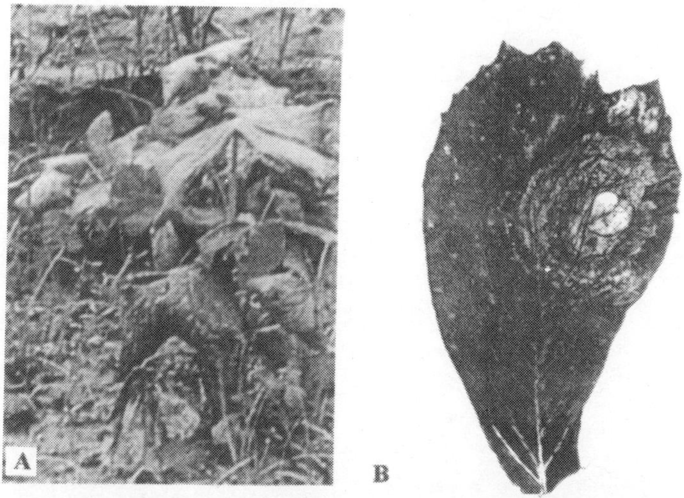

Fig. 50 : Leaf spot disease of *P. peltatum* caused by *S. podophyllina* (A) infected plant (B) infected leaflet showing typical symptoms

2. Leaf Blotch

Due to the introduction of *P. peltatum* this leaf blotch disease arrived on the European continent. The disease was not of much economic significance but found serious threat to poplar species.

Symptoms : Large spots occur on leaves causing die-back of leaves and premature leaf-fall. On the leaf spots pustules (sporodochia) with hyaline conidia appear which cause the spread of the disease to neighbouring leaves and plants (Germmen, 1987).

Causal organism : *Septotinia podophyllina* Whetzel.

14
RAUVOLFIA

The genus *Rauvolfia* was named in honour of a sixteenth century German Physician and botanist Leonard Rauvolfia. *Rauvolfia serpentina* Benth. is indigenous to India and the neighbouring countries. The plant is generally found in the moist regions with annual rainfalls of 150-375 cm and altitudes upto 1200 meters in India, Pakistan, Burma, Thailand, Sri Lanka, Malaya and Indonesia. Over 175 species of *Rauvolfia* are found in tropical and subtropical regions of the world. *Rauvolfia serpentina* grows in a wide range of climatic conditions. However, hot and humid tropical regions with sufficient rainfall are most suited places where it grows luxuriantly. *Rauvolfia serpentina* is an erect, small perennial shrub or under shrub about 60-90 cm in height. Leaves are single, thin, in whorl of three, usually crowded at the apex of the stem. Root is long, single, rarely branched, thick and gradually apexing to the base (Husain, 1993).

Although a number of species of *Rauvolfia* are reported to contain medicinally important alkaloids, only two species of *Rauvolfia* namely *Rauvolfia serpentina* Benth ex Kurz and *Rauvolfia vomitoria* Atz are commercially important and used for the production of therapeutically important alkaloids. Few drugs have attracted such a worldwide attention as the roots of *R. serpentina*. This is one of those medicinal plants which had been used in India for more than 4000 years. It was used in folk medicine even in prevedic period. In Ayurvedic system of medicine it was used for centuries in India. In Ayurveda it was used for the treatment of snake-bite, insect sting and mental disorders. It was also used for the treatment of epilepsy, diarrhoea and dysentry. Based on the Ayurvedic literature and folk medicine, chemical investigation of this palnt were taken up. *Rauvolfia* roots were reported to have potent hypotensive and tranquilizer properties. However, the main hypotensive alkaloid, reserpine was isolated by Muller and co-workers in 1952. There after rauvolfia alkaloids were adopted to modern medicine as effective hypotensive and transquilizer agent. More than 50 alkaloids have been reported from *R. serpentina*. The most important alkaloids used in medicine are reserpine, rescinnamine and desperdine. Reserpine is used as hypotensive agent as well as tranquilizer, desperdine and rescinnamine are also used as hypotensive and tranquilizer. Ajmaline, a major alkaloid of *R. serpentina* produces no sedation. Ajmaline has antifibrillar activity and is used as antiarrhythmic agent in cardiac arrhythmia.

Most of the supply of this plant is from wild sources. The plant is cultivated only in small scale in India and Bangladesh. *Rauvolfia serpentina* is susceptible to several diseases caused by fungi and viruses.

1. Wilt

The wilt disease of *R. serpentina* was first obsrved in Jammu. Since, its first appearance the disease became more and more important, because it caused considerable damage to the crop.

Symptoms : Initial symptoms of the disease consist of wilting of branches followed by wilting the entire plant. In advance stages, collar region and the root portion below the ground level turned into dark colour. Two year old plants were affected mostly. The distintegration of root cortex was more prominent in the seedling and young plant (Janardhanan *et.al.*, 1964). The foliage symptoms are characterized by dropping of leaves followed by upward curling. As the disease symptoms advanced, the entire plant was affected resulting in drying of the leaves and death of the plant.

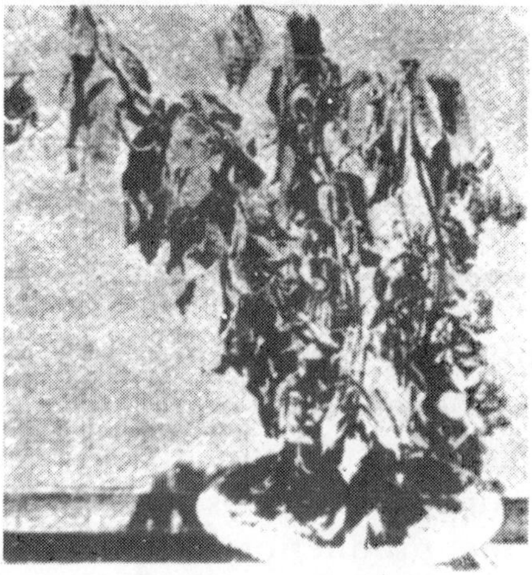

Fig. 51 : Symptoms of wilt of *R. serpentina* caused by *F. oxysporum* f. *rauvolfii*

Causal organism : Fusarium oxysporum f. sp. *rauvolfii* (Schlecht) Janardhanan, Ganguly & Husain. Mycelium extentive and cottony, pinkish-white in colour, both macro and micro condia present. Macroconidia are borne on branched conidiophores or on sporodochia mostly 2-3 septate, rarely 1 or 4 septate, hyaline, falcate 17.2-34.x2.5x4.9 μm (25.3x3.8 μm). Microconidia are generally abundant, borne on simple phiallides or rarely branched conidiophores, one – two celled, hyaline, ovoid or slightly elongated, 2.5-19.7x1.2-4.9 μm (8.1x3.4 μm). Chlamydospores terminal and intercalary globose one-celled, often present in macro-conidia. The pathogen is a

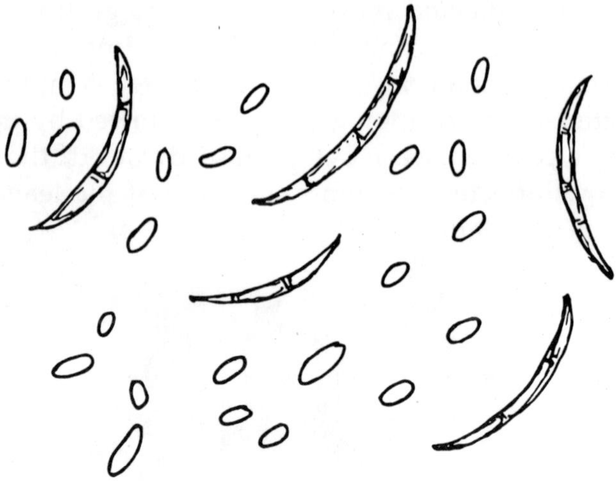

Fig. 52 : *F. oxyporum* f. *rauvolfii* : microconidia and macroconidia

new form of *F. oxysporum*, designated as *Fusarium oxysporum* f. sp. *ravoulfii* Janardhanan, Ganguly & Husain.

The pathogen was found to produce significant amount of hydrolytic enzymes *in vitro*. The host tissue stimulated the production of pectolytic enzymes (Janardhanan and Husain, 1969). The production of these enzymes was considered responsible for the extensive disintegration of the host tissue during pathogenesis. No control measures of the disease has been reported.

2. Powdery Mildew

The disease was found prevalent on *R. serpentina* in the plantations in India (Ganguly and Pandotra, 1962). The characteristic symptom of the disease was rolling of infected leaves enclosing the lower surface of the leaves which is covered with whitish growth of the fungus in patches, consisting of conidia and conidiophores. Cleistothecia are not found in natural conditions.

Causal organism : Leveillula taurica (Lev) Atz.

Control : The disease can be controlled by one application of any wettable sulphur preparation (0.3%) or Karathane WD 0.05% at the time of first appearance of the disease (Pandey, 1995).

3. Leaf Blight and Bud Rot

A leaf blight and bud rot of *R. serpentina* was frequently observed in the experimental plants. The attack is more common on one year old plants. In general the disease has been reported to be destructive in young plantations (Ganguly and Pandotra, 1962).

Symptoms : Intially small brownish circular spots with yellowish margin on the ventral surface of the tender leaves appeared. These spots then enlarged forming large dark brownish circular lesions. The spots covered the entire leaf, resulting in blight symptoms and subsequently leaves died and dropped. In certain cases young and tender portions of the tip of the branches are also infected

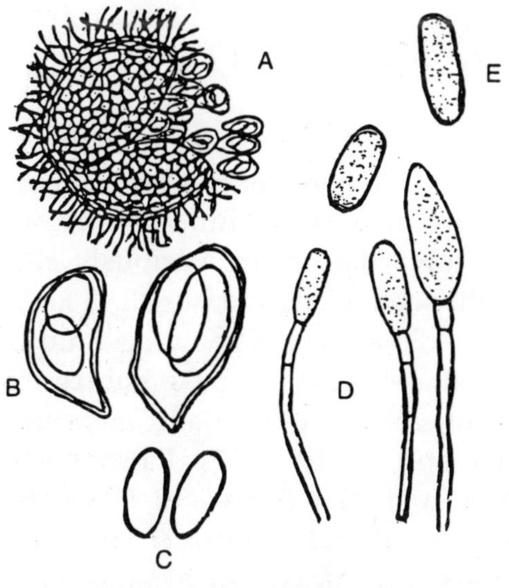

Fig. 53 : *L. taurica* (A) cleistothecium (B) asci (C) ascospores (D) conidiophores (E) conidia

leading to death of auxilliary buds. The portion of stem just below the affected leaf bud turned purplish black. Young flower buds and even the fruits are also affected (Ganguly and Pandotra, 1962).

Causal organism: Alternaria tenuis Nees.

(Syn: *Alternaria alternata* (Fr) Keissler).

Control : The disease can be controlled by spraying the infected plants with Dithane M-45 (0.3%) (Pandey, 1995). Use of seed treatment with fungicides also reduced the infection to a great extent.

4. Leaf Spots

The leaf spot disease of *R. serpentina* was first reported by Mohanty and Addy (1957) and then by Chandra (1957). The disease appeared as minute yellow spots which gradually increased in size and became dark brown patches. First purple coloured blotches appeared on the ventral surface of the leaves. In about a week's time the infected portions became dark brown in colour. The affected leaves dried and fell off (Mohanty and Addy, 1957).

Causal organism : Cercospora rauvolfiae Chupp & Muller. The conidiophores of the fungus occur in dense groups. They are pale to medium dark brown in colour, more narrow towards the tip, variously curved, rarely branched, multi-septate and measure 3.45 x 10-68 µm. The conidia are pale olivaceous in colour, cylindric, straight to slightly curved, 1-5 septate, base subtruncate to long obconically truncate, tip obtuse and measure 2.7 x 15-60 µm (Mohanty and Addy, 1957). Pandotra and Husain (1966) reported a similar disease of *R. serpentina* caused by *Cercospora serpentina* Pandotra & Husain.

Second leaf spot disease of *R. serpentina* was found to be prevalent on one year old forest nurseries (Mehrotra and Thapar, 1990). The infection caused large, irregular greenish brown spots. The tissues in the infected portion were macerated. The fungus developed a blue brown sclerotia on infected leaves. Infected leaves invariably fell off. Heavily infected plants showed defoliation to the extent of 50-70 per cent.

Causal organism : Rhizoctonia solani Khun.

Third leaf blight disease of *R. serpentina* was observed in 4 year old plantations in Madhya Pradesh (India) (Mehrotra, 1976). The pathogen attacked the leaves usually at the apex and occasionally at margins. Lower leaves were attacked first and the disease progressed upward. The fungus sporulated on the upper surface of leaves and produced dark brown to black pycnidia scattered irregularly on the infected portions. However, the diseased portions often curved upwards and became brittle towards the margins. The disease was not of much significance since only small areas of the leaves were involved.

Causal organism : Phomopsis sethii Mehrotra. Pycnidia dark-brown to black ostiolate, slightly breaked, partially embeded in the host tissue, 68.0-231.0 x 68.0-217 μm mostly 108.0-204 μm, pycnidiospores are of only one type; hyaline to subhyaline, guttulate, fusiform to oval, produced in large numbers and released in cirrus, 5.4-10.0 x 1.5-3.1 μm.

Another leaf blight of *R. serpentina* was found prevalent in the plantations in Madhya Pradesh (India) (Mehrotra, 1976). The leaf blight symptoms covered relatively larger leaf surface. The earliest symptom was a small dark roundish to angular speck on the leaves. The tiny spots, normally one or two, on the leaf at the apex alongwith the margins widened rapidly and as the disease advanced, major part of the leaf was attacked by the pathogen. Under favourable conditions the entire leaf was affected by the pathogen. The well developed spots having irregular margins showed two zones of grey and brown yellow shades. The diseased leaves became weak, pale and gradually dried up. The fungus usually sporulated heavily and produced innumerable light brown to brownish-black pycnidia on the upper surface of the leaves. The fungus was also found associated with inflorescence and drying and dead branches.

Causal organism : Macrophomina phaseolina (Tussi) Goid.

Pycnidia light brown to dark brown ostiolate, partially embedded in the host tissue, 88.4-136.0 x 88.4-122.4 µm, mostly 95.2-115.6 µm pycniospores hyaline, oval to elliptical 19.2-30.7x7.7-10.0 µm, sclerotia black of various shapes and 27.2-119.0 x 27.2-88.4 µm in size, mostly 54.4 x 95.5 x 54.4-81.6 µm.

Plantations in Madhya Pradesh (India) was also found to be affected by another leaf blight disease (Mehrotra, 1976). The pathogen persisted for relatively longer period and produced greyish-black leaf spots with pycnidia deeply seated in the infected tissue. Lower leaves were attacked first and the disease progressed upwards. The spots appeared on the leaves as inconspicuous greyish-black small area that gradually became well defined greyish-black spots. Normally, the leaves were found to bear 2-6 spots and occasionally as many as 14-18 spots were encountered. The spots were distributed all over the leaf surface and often coalesced. The spots were surrounded by a chlorotic zone. The infection caused severe defoliation.

Causal organism : Mycosphaerella rauvolfiae Ramker & Ramker. Pycnidia light brown to dark brown, ostiolate, wholly embedded in the host tissue, 34.0-81.6x34.0-78.4 µm mostly 47.6-68.0 µm; pycnidiospores hyaline, subhyaline, oval to cylindrical released in cirrus, 5.4-15.4x1.5-3.8 μm (Mehrotra, 1976).

5. Target Spot

Rauvolfia serpentina was reported to suffer heavily due to target spot disease (Mohanty and Addy, 1958, Reddy *et.al.*, 1971). The disease caused premature defoliation.

Symptoms : The leaves are attacked on both surfaces. The infection resulted in the appearance of small brownish spots which gradually enlarged into circular spots, 2-20 μm diameter with concentric zones due to which the disease is called as 'target spots'. The spots were dark brown on the upper and yellowish brown on the lower surface and are usually surrounded by a pale yellow margin. The lower leaves are infected first, the disease then progressed to upwards. Defoliation of infected plants occurred leaving behind only a few top tender leaves.

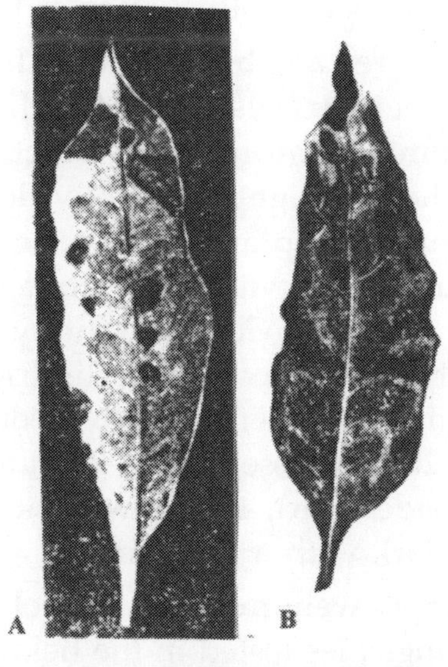

Fig. 54 : Leaf spots of *R. serpentina* (A) caused by *C. cassiicola* (B) caused by *C. rauvolfia*

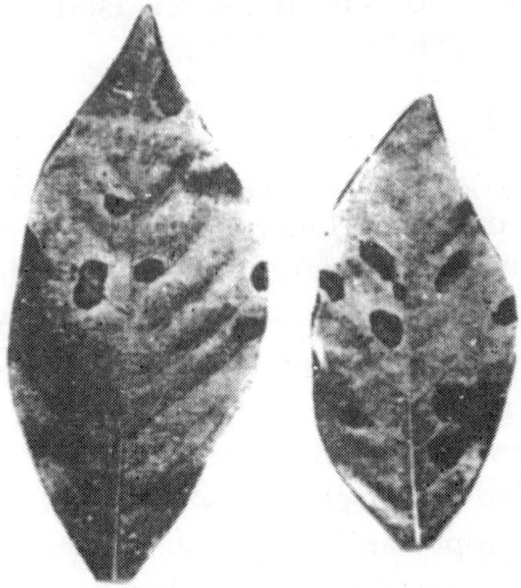

Fig. 55 : Leaf spot of *R. serpentina* caused by *M. rauvolfiae*

Causal organism : *Corynespora cassiicola* (Berk & Curt) Wei. Conidiophores arise from the mycelium emerging through the epidermis of the leaf. They occur mostly singly or sometimes in clusters on both surface of the leaf.

Colonies effuse, grey and brown, thinly hairy and the conidiophores appear iridescent. Mycelium mostly immersed; no stroma. Conidiophores erect, simple or occasionally branched, straight or slightly flexuous, pale to mid brown, smooth, septate, monoteric, percurrent with up to nine successive cylindrical proliferations, 110-850 μm long, 4-11 μm thick. Conidia solitary or catenate, very variable in shape, obclavate to cylindrical, straight or curved, subhyaline to rather pale olivaceous brown or brown, smooth, 4-20 pseudoseptate, 4-220 μm long, 9-22 μm thick in the broadest part, 4-8 μm wide at the truncate base, hilum often dark with a light rim.

Control : Attempts were made to control the disease. Among the four fungicides tested in the field, application of 0.25% Captan at monthly intervals for six months effectively controlled the disease (Reddy *et.al.*, 1971).

6. Anthracnose

Symptoms : The symptoms consist of numerous spots and the acervulli scattered all over the leaf. Infection is mainly confined to upper surface of the leaves. The spots enlarged into large circular patches and invaded the surrounding tissues. Severely infected leaves dried resulting in defoliation (Varadarajan, 1964).

Causal organism : Colletotrichum gleosporioides (Penz) Sacc.

Control : The disease is reported to be controlled by removing infected shoots and avoiding excess watering. Spraying with fermate, Dithane Z-78 and Terlate is also recommended for the control (Varadarajan, 1964).

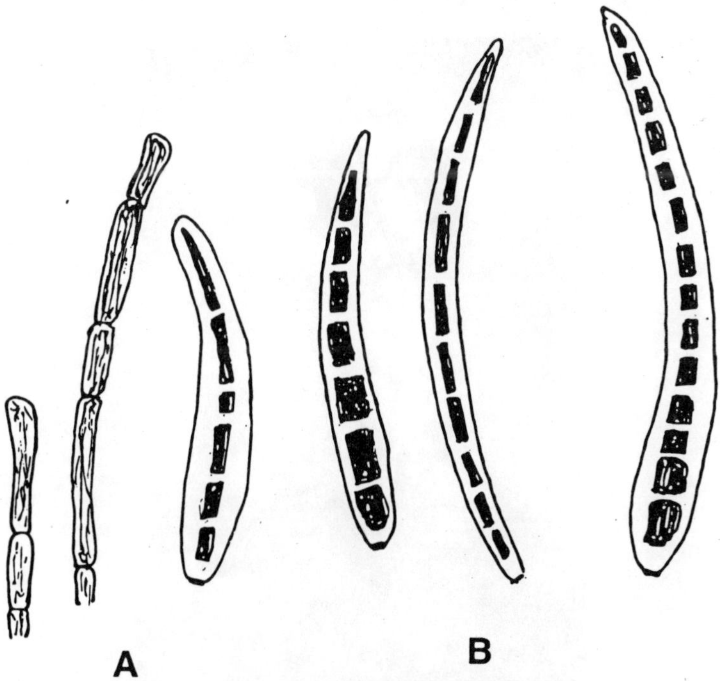

Fig. 56 : *C. cassicola* : conidiophores and conidia (A) conidiophores (B) conidia

7. Die-back

Rauvolfia serpentina has been reported to be affected by a die-back disease. The disease affected the twigs and flowers.

Symptoms : Numerous tiny spots found on leaves and stem. Acervuli are scattered all over the surface. Smaller lesions coalesced to form large and circular necrotic patches. Severe infection resulted in drying, defoliation and decapitation (Lele and Ashram, 1968, Varadarajan, 1958).

Causal organism : *Colletotrichum dematium* : (Pers) Grove.

Control : The disease is reported to be controlled by spraying the infected plants with Dithane Z-78 (0.2%). In

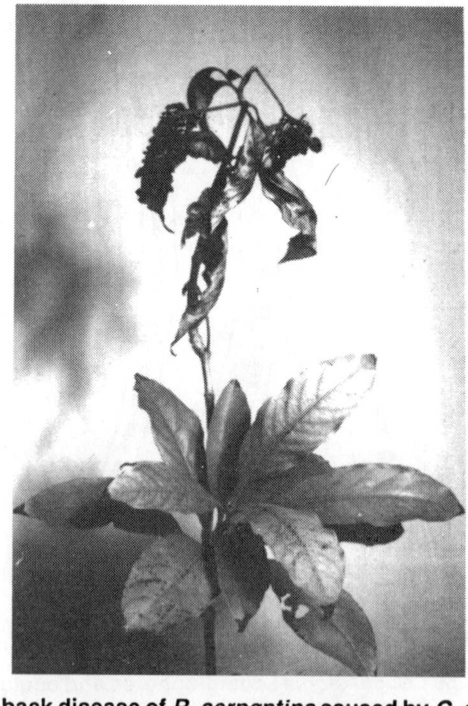

Fig. 57 : Die-back disease of *R. serpentina* caused by *C. dematium*

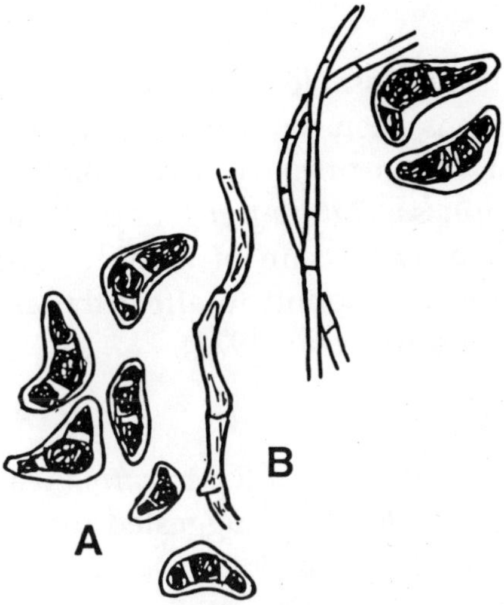

Fig. 58 : *C. lunata* : conidia and conidiophores (A) conidia (B) conidiophores

the advance stage of infection pruning of infected parts is recommended.

A leaf spot disease and premature defoliation of *R. serpentina* was observed on cultivated plants in Gujarat (India). The symptoms consisted of severe leaf spots and defoliation (Varadarajan, 1966).

Causal organism : *Curvularia lunata* (Wakker) Boed. Conidia are arranged at the tip of conidiophores, pale brown, thin septate, third cells from the base larger and darker than others, unequally ventricose to fusiform and measuring 23.4-39.0 x 7.8-15.6 μm (28.6 x 10.4 μm). Spores spirally arranged in whorls. Spores have only three septa with a single cell usually third from the base being disproportionally large. End cells of the conidia tend to remain more or less hyaline and hilum inserted.

Control : Two to three sprayings a week with Bordeaux mixture for 4-6 weeks are reported to control the disease.

8. Mosaic

A sap transmissable virus causing mosaic disease of *R. serpentina* has been reported. The virus produced local necrotic lesions on primary leaves of *Phaseolus vulgaris, Nicotiana glutinosa, Datura metel* and *D. innoxia*. The virus was identified as a strain of tobacco mosaic virus. The virus infection was found to affect the alkaloid contents of the roots (Sastry *et.al.*, 1973).

9. Phyllody

Bunchy top disease of *R. serpentina* was first observed by Varadarajan (1967). He suggested the overwintering of the disease in *Catharanthus roseus, Nicotiana tabacum, Solanum melongena* and *Capsicum annum* in Gujarat (India). A disease with similar symptoms was observed in 1964

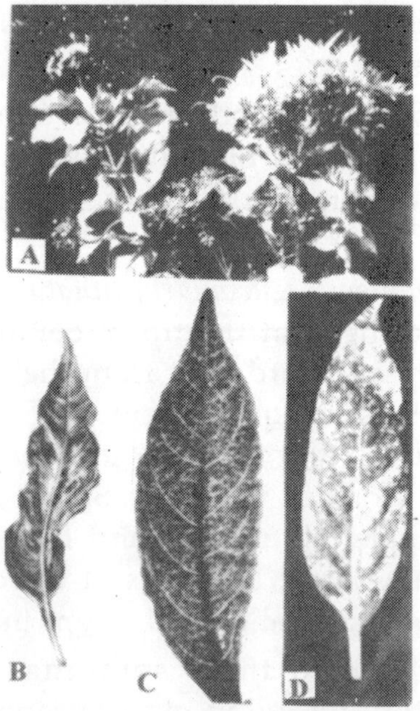

Fig. 59 : Symptoms of different viral diseases of *R. serpentina* (A) phyllody (B) mosiac (C) yellow vein (D) ring spot

in Jammu (Sastry, 1973). The disease was found transmitted to *Rauvolfia* by grafting and by stem parasite (*Cuscuta* sp).

Symptoms : Characteristic symptoms of the disease were retarded growth, shortened internodes, phyllody of flowers. The leaves became small and pale in colour; the floral parts of the infected plants are modified to leaf like structures resulting into a cluster of small leaves in place of inflorescence and leading to complete sterility. The disease was found to appear on all branches or any one flowering branch of the plant. The disease adversely affected the alkaloid content of the plant (Sastry, 1973). The disease is probably caused by a virus resembling Aster yellow virus.

10. Yellow Vein Mosaic

A yellow vein disease of *R. serpentina* caused by a graft transmissable and whitefly (*Bemisia tabaci*) transmitted virus, was observed in the experimental plantations in Jammu.

Symptoms : The symptoms consisted of yellowing of young leaves and formation of yellow network in the back ground of green surface. A minor retardation of growth of infected plants was also observed. Reduction in root biomass and total alkaloid contents of roots occurred due to the disease (Sastry, 1973).

11. Ring Spot

A graft transmissable ring spot disease of *R. serpentina* was observed in the experimental plantations in Jammu.

Symptoms : Leaves of infected plants showed characteristic concentric yellow rings of different sizes scattered all over the surface of the leaves. The rings gradually enlarged, coalesced and became gradually necrotic. In later stages, the entire infected leaves became necrotic resulting in defoliation. Infection adversely affected the quality of roots and their alkaloid contents (Sastry, 1973).

12. Green Mosaic

Rauvolfia serpentina was reported to be affected by a severe green mosaic virus. The diseased plants showed severe stunting and the leaves narrowed. Mosaic mottling sympotoms were more pronounced in young leaves (Sastry, 1973).

Causal organism : The virus was identified as a strain of cucumber mosaic virus (CMV). The virus was isometric, 27 nm in diameter and was transmitted by aphid (*Myzus persica*) but not by seeds or soil. Mode of transmission, host range, biophysical properties and serological relationship showed that the virus is an isolate of Cucumber mosaic virus (CMV).

13. Root-Knot

Infected roots were covered with galls of various sizes from small dot to 8 mm diameter. They are present on roots even upto 6 feet depth. The infected plants showed stunted growth, etiolation and smaller leaves. The disease was reported to be caused by a nematode, *Meloidogyne incognita* (Kofoid & White) Chitwood (Haseeb *et.al.*, 1983).

Control : Soil fumigation, adoption of proper cultural practices and development of resistant variaties are useful methods for the control of diseases caused by nematodes.

15
SENNA

Dried leaves and pods of *Cassia angustifolia* Vahl is known in commerce as Indian senna and that of *Cassia acutifolia* Delile as Alexandrian senna. Senna was used by Arab physicians as early as 900 A.D. The Arabs introduced this in South India by the traders. *Cassia angustifolia* is indigenous to Somalia, Southern Arabia, Sind and Kutch area in India. The plant is mainly cultivated in the Southern districts of Tamil Nadu in India. *Cassia acutifolia* is indigenous to Sudan and Sinai. It is cultivated in Sudan and Egypt. *Cassia angustifolia* is a small, perennial, erect undershrub and C. *acutifolia* is a semi-herbaceous shrub. The two species are very similar in morphology. Senna leaves and pods contain anthraquinone glycosides, the important ones are Sennoside A and B used in medicine. In addition, Sennoside C and D have been isolated. In modern medicine Sennosides are used as calcium sennoside tablets. Sennosides are laxative. In traditional medicine, an infusion of leaves in the form of tea is used as laxative (Husain, 1993).

Senna (*Cassia angustifolia* and *Cassia acutifolia*) are affected by a number of diseases. Damping-off, leaf spots and leaf blights are the major diseases of this crop.

1. Damping-off

Damping-off affecting the seedlings is the most devastating disease of this crop. The disease is common on most of the soils in North-west India where this crop is cultivated. The disease spreads fast, if the drainage is insufficient.

Symptoms : The infected plants showed blackening on the collar region extending upwards leading to death of seedlings. Infection caused death of plants in patches in the field (Patel and Patel, 1984).

Causal organism : *Macrophomina phaseolina* (Tassi) Goid (*Syn: Rhizoctonia bataticola* (Taub) Butler). Sclerotia within roots, black, smooth, hard 100 μm-1 mm dia (in culture 50-300 μm). Pycnidia dark brown, solitary, immersed becoming erumpent, 100-200 μm dia, opening by apical ostioles, pycnidial wall multicellular with heavily pigmented thick-walled cells on the outermost side. Conidiophores hyaline short obpyriform to cylindrical, 5-13x4-6 μm. Conidia hyaline, ellipsoid to obovoid 14-30 x 5-10 μm. The pathogen has wide spread distribution in tropics and sub-tropics.

Control : Treating the seeds with Thiran or Captan (2.5 g/kg) protects the growing seedlings from the disease. Drenching the field with Bavistin (0.1%) Brassicol (0.2%) or Rhizoctol (0.1-0.5%) is beneficial to delimit the disease or partially control the infection. It is advisable not to grow senna again in the same field where infection was observed earlier.

2. Leaf Blight

Symptoms : Leaf blight disease has been reported to cause serious damage to senna crop. Initial symptoms are minute, dark brown circular spots on the laminae especially at the tip and margins of the leaflets. The spots enlarged to 3-8 μm turned brown to black in colour and became irregular. Chlorotic areas from the tip and margins were found to spread over the entire leaf blade leading to drying and premature leaf fall. Older leaves were more

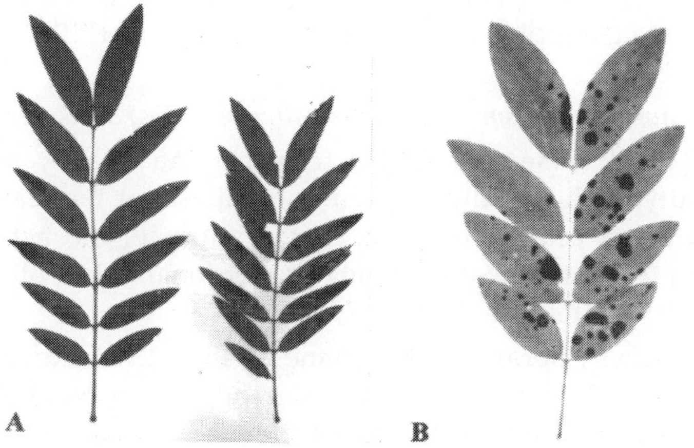

Fig. 60 : Leaf blight disease caused by (A) *A. alternata* (B) *G. cingulata*

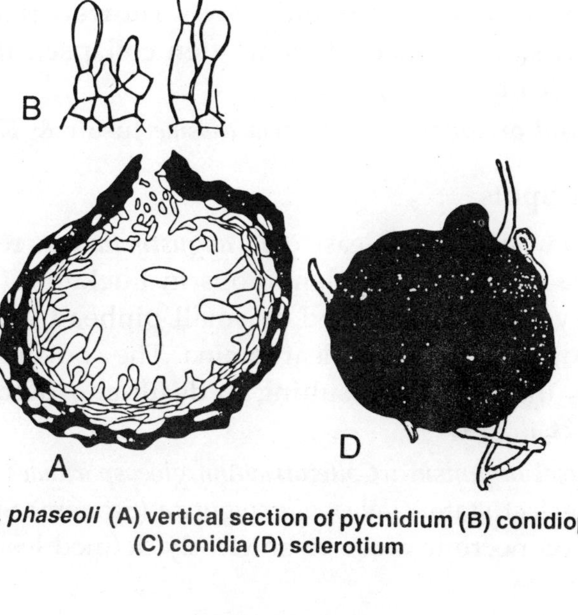

Fig. 61 : *M. phaseoli* (A) vertical section of pycnidium (B) conidiophores (C) conidia (D) sclerotium

susceptible to infection than young ones. *Cassia acutifolia* was less susceptible compared to *C. angustifolia* (Pillai and Patel 1982).

Causal organism : Alternaria alternata (Fr.) Keissler.

The disease was found to affect the quality and quantity of the produce. Chemical analysis of the leaves of infected plants revealed that sennoside, the active principle, content was inversely proportional to leaf blight intensity (Patel and Pillai 1979).

Control : Spraying of Dithane M-45 (0.15%) thrice at an interval of 15 days for a period of 5-6 weeks is recommended for the control of the disease.

Singh *et.al.*, (1996) reported a new leaf blight disease affecting *C. angustifolia*. The symptoms consisted of small, pale to dark brown spots that became large lesions in later stage. The lesions first appeared on the tips and margins of leaf lets and later coalesced leading to complete necrosis of leaves. The disease caused blighted appearance in the field. Dark, irregular sports were also observed on the stem and pods. Infected pods showed irregular discolourisation. Infected stem often collapsed thereby causing death of the plants.

Causal organism : Alternaria cassiae Jurair & Khan.

3. Leaf Spots

A new leaf spot disease of *C. angustifolia* was reported from the experimental plantations in Lucknow (India). Initial symptoms appeared as small pinhead brown to dark brown spots on the leaf lamina. The spots enlarged towards the margins resulting to death and defoliation (Gupta *et.al.*, 1997).

Causal organism : Colletotrichum gloeosporioides (Penz) Sacc. (perfect state: *Glomerella cingulata* (Stonem) Spauld). Acervli on necrotic areas or on clearly defined lesions on the leaves, usually setose, sometimes sparsely setose, glabrous, round, elongated or irregular. Setae variable in length, rarely more than 200 µm long and 4-8 µm wide, 1-4 septate, brown slightly swollen at the base and tapering to the apex on which conidia are usually borne. Conidia cylindrical sometimes slightly ellipsoide with round apex and narrow truncate base, hyaline, aseptate,

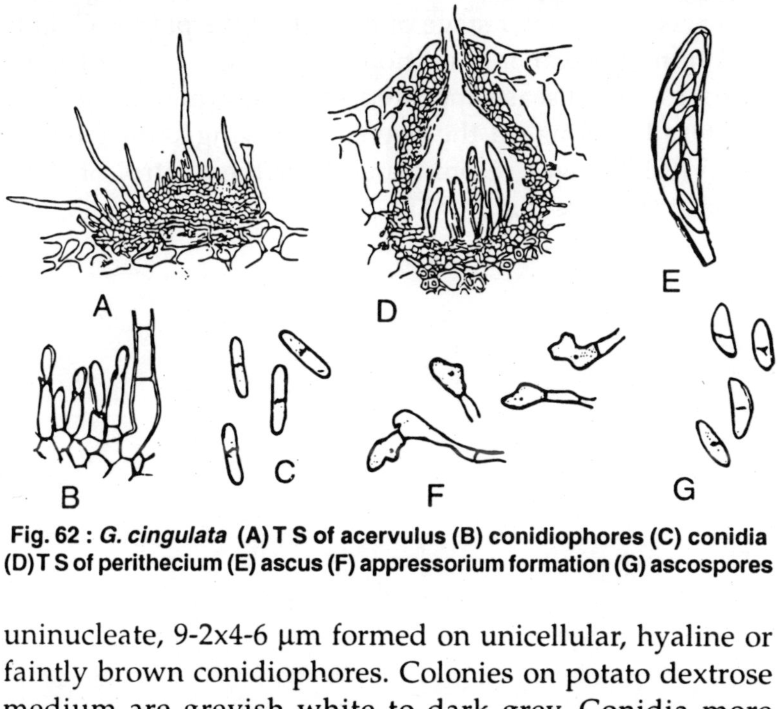

Fig. 62 : *G. cingulata* (A) T S of acervulus (B) conidiophores (C) conidia (D) T S of perithecium (E) ascus (F) appressorium formation (G) ascospores

uninucleate, 9-2x4-6 µm formed on unicellular, hyaline or faintly brown conidiophores. Colonies on potato dextrose medium are greyish white to dark grey. Conidia more variable in size and shape than in host. Perithecia occasionally formed in young cultures more common in older cultures. Appressoria formed on mycelium in old cultures. Perithecia are observed on various parts of the host, usually on dead leaves and twigs, solitary or aggregated globose to obpyriform, dark brown to black 85-300 µm dia, wall upto 8 cell thick, pseudoparenchymatous within, ostiole slightly papillate, circular, canal lined with periphyses. Asci 8 spored, clavate to cylindrical, thickened at apex, 35-80x8-14 µm interspersed with paraphyses forming group at base of the perithecium. Ascospores oval to cylindrical to fusiform, unicellular hyaline.

A number of leaf spot and leaf blight diseases of minor importance have been reported to affect senna. Leaf blights caused by *Phyllosticta* Sp and *Cercospora* Sp were observed in the later stage of growth of the plants. Cloudy and humid weather conditions favoured spread of these diseases. The disease appeared as small brown irregularly scattered lesions on the leaves. Spraying with Dithane M-45 (0.15%) was recommended for the control of these disease (Pareek *et.al.,* 1980).

16
WITHANIA

Withania somnifera Dunal is an erect, evergreen shrub distributed throughout the drier parts of India and also in the Mediterranean regions. It is cultivated on commercial scales in the central part of India. The commercial drug consists of the dried roots. Several alkaloidal and non alkaloidal compounds were isolated from *W. somnifera*. The important compounds isolated from different parts of the plant are steroidal lactones called Withanolids. Many biochemically heterogenous alkaloids have been isolated from roots. Total alkaloid fraction of roots extract of cultivated plants exhibited prolonged hypotensive, bradycardiac and respiratory stimulant activities in dogs. The total alkaloid fraction also showed relaxant and antispasmodic effectts. Withaferin A is the most important withanolids isolated so far which has potent antimicrobial activity. Withaferin A has been reported to show anticancer activity. The compound also showed potent anti-arthritic and anti-inflammatory properties. In Ayurvedic literature W. *somnifera* is referred as Ashwagandha. Its roots are prescribed for hiceup, female disorders, cough, rheumatism and as a sedative. It is useful in the treatment of inflammatory conditions, ulcers and scabies. Ashwagandha is often referred as Indian Ginseng, because of its antifatigue properties. The roots are also demonstrated to have significant psychotropic effects and antitumor activity. A number of diseases of this crop caused by fungi, viruses and phytoplasma have been reported.

1. Damping-off and Seedling-rot

Damping-off and seedling-rot mortality caused serious damage to the crop. The plant population is drastically reduced which resulted in reduced root yield.

Symptoms : The infected plants turned yellowish and finally dried up. In case of damping-off, the leaves of affected plants showed mottling followed by necrotic lesions, curling and burnt margins. In severe cases of infection whole plant was burnt and died (Pandey, 1988; Nigam, 1984; Gupta *et.al.*, 1993).

Causal organism : Alternaria alternata (Fr.) Keissler.

Control : Jain (1985) reported the use of fungicidal treatment of seeds for the control of seedling diseases. He found that Deltan, Dithane M45, Brassicol and Bavistin could protect the seedlings. Pandey (1987) tested a number of fungicides to check the seedling mortalility and found Bayletan followed by Brassicol proved most effective for seedling diseases. Nigam (1984) also reported that seedling mortality could be reduced by seed treatment with Dithane M-45 at 3g/kg seed.

Seedling mortality became serious under high temperature and humid conditions. The spread of the causal organism was very high in the months of August and September and the damage increased, if the rains followed after the sowing. The disease could be minimised by use of seeds collected from healthy plants, crop rotation, timely sowing and by keeping fields well drained.

2. Leaf Blight and Die-back

Die-back and leaf blight disease caused significant damage to Ashwagandha crop. The disease was first reported by Pandey and Nigam (1985).

Symptoms : The characteristic symptoms of the disease are the appearance of small light brown spots on leaves and flowers which enlarged, coalesced resulting in blight symptoms. In case of die-back, the disease caused necrosis of tender twigs from the tip backwards. The entire branch or the top of the plant withered. The dead twigs were greyish brown or straw coloured in the advanced stage of infection (Pandey *et.al.*, 1985).

Causal organism : *Alternaria alternata* (Fr.) Keissler.

Control : Use of seeds from disease-free plants, spraying of the crop with fungicides, such as Dithane M-45 (0.3%) or Rovaral (0.2%) have been found to check the spread of the disease. Seed dressings by suitable fungicides has also been found to control the disease to a large extent during the early stage (Pandey *et.al.*, 1985).

3. Leaf Spot

The disease was reported from Jaipur, India (Mahrishi, 1986). The disease appeared during the rainy season.

Symptoms : Symptoms were small dirty yellow to brown coloured, water soaked spots with a violet periphery and chlorotic halo on the leaves. The spots enlarged coalesced and became brittle. Sporodochia of the fungus were observed in the lower surface of the infected leaves.

Causal organism : *Myrothecium roridum* Tode ex Fies. Sporodochia sessile or rarely stipitate, polymorphic in surface view; size variable, diameter 16-750 (258) μm, depth 50-200 (70) μm. Spore mass wet when young, drying hard, shiny black, convex, surrounded by a fringe of entangled white hyphae. Marginal hyphae controted, hyaline, usually tapering towards a blunt apex, branched, septate, cells 20-30 x 1-2.2 μm. No external mycelium

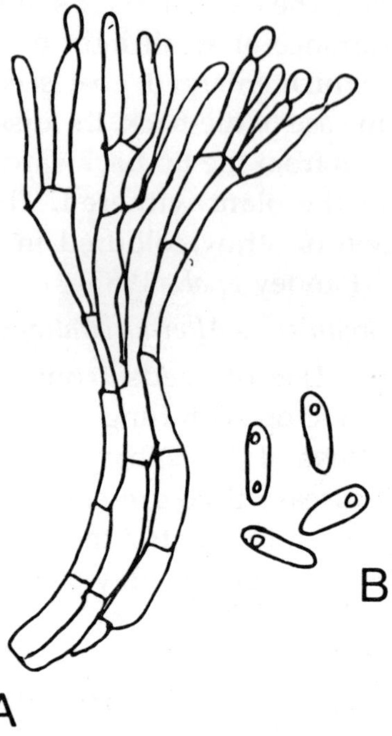

Fig. 63 : *M. roridum* : (A) conidiophores (B) conidia

found on plant material. Conidiophores arising directly from the mycelium in culture or from the epidermal cells of the host where the basal cells of the conidiophores are short, 6.3-13.5 x 1.8-2.3 µm and closely compacted forming a stromatic layer with the host epidermal cells. Conidiophores hyaline, cylindrical, branched below and then into two or three branches bearing the phialides, closely compacted together, septate, cells 6.3-23 x 1.4-3.6 µm. Phialides in whorls of two to five at apex of conidiophore branches, mostly cylindrical, rarely clavate, hyaline, some light olivaceous, occasionally the apex darkened, 9-27 x 0.9-1.8 µm closely compacted into parallel rows forming a dense layer. Sproes rod-shaped, ends rounded, one end rarely slightly truncate, smooth walled, hyaline to light olivaceous, black in mass, guttulate, 5.6-8.4 x 1.8-2.8 µm.

4. Root-knot

Among the phytonematodes, the root-knot nematodes has the widest distribution. Root-knot nematodes are reported to be responsible for the significant reduction in plant growth and yields.

Symptoms : A severe root-knot infection was observed on *W. somnifera.* Infected plants showed yellowing and stunting. Roots of infected plants showed formation of galls, swellings or knots (Bhatti *et.al.*, 1974; Minz and Harari, 1969).

Causal organism : Meloidogyne javanica (Treuk) Chitwood.

5. Leaf Curl

Phatak and Raychaudhari (1967) reported accurrence of tobacco leaf curl virus on *W. somnifera.* Symptoms of the disease were vein clearing, curling, puckering and occasionally rolling. The surface of infected leaves was wrinkled. Some leaves were malformed.

Causal organism : Tobacco leaf curl virus.

6. Witches' Broom

A witches broom disease of *W. somnifera* was reported from Lucknow, India. The disease first appeared in the experimental plantations. The disease then spread to commercial fields causing considerable damage.

Symptoms : Typical symptoms of the disease were small leaves, shortening of internodes, excessive branching resulting in witches broom appearance, premature drying and death of infected twigs and leaves. Infected plants remained stunted. Ultra-thin sections of infected leaf tissue showed pleomorphic bodies, measuring 250-550 nm, in the sieve tubes of phloem and the disease was transmitted from infected plants to healthy plants through

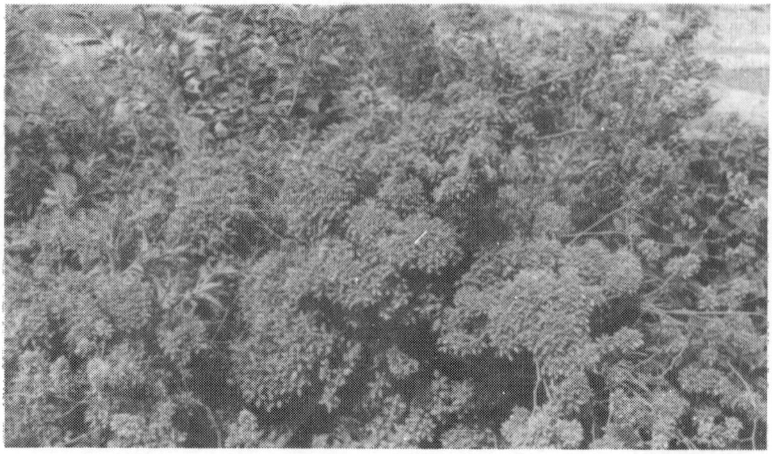

Fig. 64 : Symptoms of witch's broom or phyllody of *W. somnifera* caused by *Phytoplasma* (Courtesy of Dr. M. Zaim, CIMAP, Lucknow)

grafting. Treatment of infected plants with tetracycline gave temporary recovery from typical symptoms of the disease after 15-20 days of treatment (Zaim and Samad, 1995).

Causal organism : Phytoplasma (Mycoplasma-like organism). Pleomorphic bodies present in the sieve tubes of phloem. The bodies are generally oval/spherical, variable in size ranging between 250-550 nm. They were densely stained and of high electron-opacity and bound by unit membrane. Occasionally found to undergo budding. The organism is highly sensitive to tetracyclines.

Control : Spray with tetracyclines has been recommended for the control of the disease. The recovery of the disease symptoms is often temporary.

BIBLIOGRAPHY

Abraham, Z., Srivastava, A.K. and Bagchi, G.D. 1988. Cytoplasmic vesicles containing secondary metabolites in the roots of *Coleus forskohlii* (Willd.) Briq. *Curr. Sci.* **57** : 1337-1339.

Alam, M., Sattar, A., and Janardhanan, K.K., 1998. Management of damping-off disease of opium poppy. *Indian Phytopath.* **51** : 269-272.

Alam, M., Sattar, A., Chourasia, H.K., and Janardhanan, K.K. 1996. Damping-off, a new disease of opium poppy caused by *Pythium dissotocum. Indian Phytopath* **49** : 94-97.

Alavi, A., 1975. How to prevent and control downy mildew. *Iranian. J. Plant. Path.* 73.

Alcock, N.L. 1926. A preliminary note on *A. belladonna Pharmaceutical J.* 116-232.

Anand, G.P.S. and Summanwar, A.S., 1981. Studies on a mosaic disease of opium poppy. *Indian Phytopath* **34** : 262.

Angell, H.R., 1950. Seedling blight, II. Soil in relation to seedling blight of opium poppy and peas. *Aust. J. Agric Res.* **1** : 132.

Anonymous, 1980. *Annual Report Rabi of AICRP on medicinal and aromatic plants, Anand, India.*

Anonymous, 1984. *Annual Report of All India Coordinated Research Project (M&AP)* for the year 1984-85. NBPGR, New Delhi, pp. 6-7.

Anonymous, 1988. *Report on trials sixth. All India workshop on medicinal and aromatic plants and related schemes,* presented at 23rd Agresco meeting, Gujarat Agricultural University, Anand, India.

Atanosoff. D. Dodoff, D.N., Kovacevski, I.C. Martinoff, S.I., Trifonova Mme. V. and Christoff, A., 1932. Parasitic fungi new to Bulgaria. *Third Contribution. Year Book. Univ. of Sofia, Fac. Agric, Sofia* 10 : 341-366.

Balasubramanian, K.R. and Bhama, V.S., 1977. A new leaf spot disease of *Catharanthus roseus* in India. *Indian Phytopath*, **3** : 556-557.

Ballarin, C., 1950. Studies on *Helminthosporium papaveris. Phytopath. Z.* **16:** 400.

Baruah, P., Bhuyan, P.D. and Singh, R.S. 1995. Tuber rot of steriodal *Dioscorea floribunda* Mart and Gal – a new record. *Indian Forester*,**121** : 431-432.

Batool, F. and Haseeb, A., 1996. Influence of *Glomus aggregatum* on root-knot development caused by *Meloidogyne incognita* in *Hyoscyamus muticus. Afro-Asian J. Nematol.* **6:** 188-190.

Beaumont, A., 1953. Disease of poppies. *Gdners. Chron. Ser.* **3**: 71.

Benson, D.M., 1995. Aluminium amendment of potting mixes for control of *Phytophthora* damping-off in bedding plants. *Hort Science* **30**: 1413-1416.

Bhakuni, D.S. and Jain, S., 1995. Chemistry of cultivated medicinal plants. In : *Advances in Horticulture.* Vol.11, K.L. Chadha and R. Gupta (Ed.) Malhotra Publishing House, New Delhi, p 45-119.

Bhatti, D.S., Gupta, D.C., Dahiya, R.S. and Malhan, I., 1974. Additional hosts of root-knot nematode *Meloidogyne javanica. Curr. Sci.* **43**: 622-623.

Bode, O. und Marcus, O., 1959. Untersuchungen Uber eine virose von *Atropa belladonna* L. *Verh IV. Intern. Pflanzenschutz Kongr.* Hamburg. 1957, Bd **1:** 375-376.

Bogarada, A.P. Lyman, V.E. and Taranich, A.P., 1971. On the resistance of poppy to Helminthosporiosis. *Selekts Semenov.* **36**: 78.

Boruah, P., Deka, P. and Bordoloi, D.N., 1992. Leaf blight of *Dioscorea composita* from north east India. *J. Assam Sci. Soc.* **34**: 25-27, 1992.

Butler, E.J., 1918. *Fungi and Disease in plants*, Thacker Spink & Co., Calcutta, pp.499-506.

Capoor, S.P. and Varma, P.M., 1952. Studies on the distortion mosaic virus of *Datura innoxia* Mill. *Indian J. Agri Sci.* **22**: 303-314.

Casulli, F. and Ippolito. A., 1995. Observations on liquorice rust (*Uromyces glycyrrhizae* (Rab) Magn. in South Italy. *Informatore-Fitopathologico.* **45**: 27-30.

Celino, M.S. 1934. Blight of Cinchona seedlings. *Philippine Agr.*, **23**: 111-127.

Chakravarty, D.K. , Khatua, D.C. and Dass, T.K. 1976. Pathological problems in the cultivation of *Vinca rosea. Ind. Agri.* **20**: 289-295.

Chandra, V. 1956. Studies on *Rauvolfia.* Part V: *Alternaria* on *Rauvolfia serpentina* Benth. *Ind. J. Pharm.* **18**: 146.

Chastagner, G.A. Ogawa, J.M. and Sammeta, K.P.V. 1979. Cause and control of damping-off in *Plantago ovata. Plant. Dis. Reptr.* **62**: 929-932.

Chenulu, V.V., Sachidananda, J. and Mehta, S.C. 1968. Studies on a mosaic disease of henbane (*Hyoscyamus niger* L) from India. *Indian Phytopath.* **21**: 408-415.

Cheon, S.R. and Kim. H.J. 1999. Comparison of resistance of root-rot caused by *Fusarium solani* in ginseng breeding lines. *Korean J. Ginseng Sci.* **14**: 50-56.

Chopra, R.N., Chopra, I.C., Handa, K.L. and Kapoor, L.D. *Indigenous drugs of India,* 2nd Ed. U.N. Dhar & Sons Private Ltd., Calcutta, 1958, p. 816.

Christoff, A. 1931. A bacterial blight of opium poppy *Renseignements agricoles (Sofia)* **12**: 27-46.

Christoff, A. 1933. A new bacterial blight of opium poppy caused by *Bacillus (Erwinia) papaveri n. sp. J. Agric. Exp. Stn. Sofia* **5**: 31.

Christoff, A. 1934. Some plant diseases new to Bulgaria: 2nd contribution. *Bull. Soc. Bot de Bulgaria* **6**: 37.

Chung, H.S. 1974. The status of past and present research and problems of ginseng diseases, pp. 55-67 in *Korean Ginseng Science Symposium.* Korean Society of Pharmacognosy Press, Seoul.

Cleij, G. 1961. Beet yellow in poppy. *Euphytica* **10:** 225.

Conti, G.G., Marte, M. and Leone, G. 1983. Effect of light and dark on callose deposition during the hypersensitive reaction in *Datura stramonium* infected with tobacco mosaic virus. *Rivisti di Pathologica Vegetale* **19**: 85-97.

Cook, M.T. 1939. Entermedades de las plantas economicas de las *Antillas Univ. Puerto Rico Monograph, Ser B* **4**, 530 p.

Coster, Ch. 1941. The work of West Java Research Institute, Buitenzorg, 1938-1941. *Empire Town. Exp. Agr.* **10**: 22-30.

Crandall, B.S. 1947. Cinchona root disease caused by *Phytophthora cinnamomi*. *Phytopathology*, **37**: 918-929.

Crandall, B.S. and Davis, W.C. 1944. Occurrence of cinchona root-rot in America, U.S. Dept. Agri. *Pl. Dis Reptr.* **28**: 926-929.

Crandall, B.S. and Davis, W.C. 1945. Phytophthora wilt and stem canker of cinchona. *Phytopathology* **35**, 138-140.

Dabek, A.J. 1982. Transmission experiments on coconut lethal yellowing disease with *Deltocephalus flavicostu* Stol, a leaf hopper Vector of periwinkle phyllody in Jamaica. *Phytopath. Z.* **103**: 109-119.

Dale, J.L. and Fletcher, J. 1987. First report of periwinkle infection by Mycoplasma like organism from field collected blueberry leaf hoppers. *Plant Dis.* **71**: 1045.

Darley, E.F. and Flores. M.A. 1951. Two cankers of Cinchona in Guatemala caused by *Phytophthora cinnamomi* and *P. parasitica. Phytopathology* **41** : 641-647.

Darmono, T.W. and Parke, J.L. 1990. Chlamydospores of *Phytophthora cactorum*: their production, structure and infectivity. *Can. J. Bot.* **68**: 640-645.

Darmono, T.W. Own, M.L. and Parke, J.L. 1991. Isolation and pathogenicity of *Phytophthora cactorum* from forest and ginseng garden soil in Wisconsin. *Plant Dis.* **75**: 610-612.

Darpouse, H. 1945. A contribution to the study of the diseases of oleogenous plants in France *Ann. Epiphyt. N.S.* **11:** 71.

Davino, O., Urso, F.D. and Carbone, M. 1993. Discovery of tomato spotted wilt tospovirus (TSMV) on periwinkle in Sicily. *Tecnica Agricole* **45**: 127-135.

De Souza, N.J. 1991. *Coleus forskohlii* Briq–the Indian plant source for forskolin. In: *Recent Advances in Medicinal, Aromatic & Spice Crops,* **Vol 1:** (Ed. S.P. Raychaudhuri) pp. 83-91.

Desai, M.V. and Desai, D.S. 1969. Control of downy mildew of isabgul by aurofungin. *Hindustan Antibiotic Bull* **1**: 254-257.

Deshpande, A.L. Agarwal, J.P. and Mathur, B.N. 1969. *Rhizoctonia bataticola* causing root-rot of opium in Rajasthan. *Indian Phytopath.* **22:** 510-511.

Dobos, J. 1988. Possibilities of protection against *Septoria digitalis* Pass. *Herba Hungarica,* **27**: 81-88.

Doshi, A. and Thakore, B.B.L. 1995. Effect of fungicidal seed treatment on primary infection of downy mildew and viability of opium seeds. *Ind. J. Mycol. Plant Pathol* **25:** 160-164.

Doshi, A. and Thakore, B.B.L. 1995. Influence of host nutrition on the development of downy mildew disease of opium poppy. *Indian Phytopath.* **48:** 335-338.

Dyer, R.A. 1949. Botanical surveys and control of plant diseases. *Fmg. S. Afr.* **24:** 119.

El-Hammady, M., Shatla, M.N. and El-Khalwagy. M.H. 1977. Virus diseases of some medicinal plants in Egypt II CMV and PVX on *Datura stramonium* L. *Agri. Res. Rev.* **55**: 145-155.

Ernwein, C. and Wetter. C. 1987. Ultrastructure of inclusions formed by ribgrass mosaic virus in leaf cells. *J. Phytopathology,* **119**: 216-224.

Felklova, M. 1977. Pathophysiological study of some diseases of medicinal plants. *Referativnyi Zhurnal Biologiya* **7G**: 406.

Fenne, S.B., 1942. *Cercospora* on belladonna in Virginia. *Plant Dis. Reptr.* **26**: 280.

Fokin, A.D. 1922. Diseases and injuries of cultivated plants observed during the summer of 1922 in the Govt of Vyatka. *Trans. Fourth All Russian Entomo. Phytopath. Congress Moscow,* 8-14 Dec., 1922, p.108.

Gahukar, K.B. and Patil, J.B. 1991. Identification of viruses inciting mosaic in Datura. *PKV Res. J.* **15**: 45-48.

Ganguly, D. and Pandotra, V.R. 1962. *Regional Research Laboratory, Jamm. Bull.* **1**: 42-46.

Ganguly, D. and Pandotra, V.R. 1962. Some commonly occurring diseases of important medicinal and aromatic plants in Jammu and Kashmir. *Indian Phytopath,* **15**: 50-54.

Ganguly, D. and Pandotra, V.R. 1963. Fungi on medicinal and aromatic plants in the north west Himalayas. I. *Mycopath. Mycol. appl.* **20**: 39-48.

Gill. H.S., Riberio. O.K. and Zentmeyer, G.A. 1977. *Phytophthora* blight of periwinkle in Cochella valley of California. *Plant. Dis. Reptr.* **61**: 560-561.

Giorgodze. R.D. 1989. Virus causing mosaic of periwinkle. *Zaschita Rasteini* (Moskva) **3**: 30-31.

Girzitska, Mme. Z.K. 1928. Condial stage of *Pleospora papaveracea Sacc. Protc. Pan. Soviet Congress Botanists* Leningrad, January 1928. p.172.

Goto, U. 1938. Anthracnose of *Digitalis* caused by *Colletotrichum fuscum* Laubert. *Ann. Phytopath Soc. Japan* **8**: 1-8.

Goyal, R. and Pathak, N.C. 1982. A new leaf spot disease of *Catharanthus roseus* (L) G. Don from India. *New Botanist* **9**: 31-32.

Gremmen, J. 1987. Notes on the mayapple and the life history of the fungus *Septotinia podophyllina. Mycotaxon* **28**: 255-256.

Grimaldi, V. and Grasso, S. 1988. Mycoplasma disease of *Dineorphotheca sinuata* and *Catharanthus roseus* in Sicily. *Acta-Horticulturae* **234**: 137-143.

Grummer, G. 1953. The influence of *Alternaria* infection of poppy capsules on promptitude of germination by their seeds. *Flora Fauna.* **140**: 298.

Grzybowska, T. 1976. The pathogenicity of isolates of *Septoria digitalis* Pass and the susceptibility to them of foxglove species. *Rocznik. Nauk. Rolniczych,* **6:** 165-182.

Gupta, M.L., Janardhanan, K.K. and Husain, A. 1986. Fusarium root-rot of opium poppy. *FAO Plant. Prot. Bull.* **34**: 108-109.

Gupta, M.L., Janardhanan, K.K. 1989. A new leaf blight of opium poppy caused by *Alternaria pharmagmospora* van Emden. *Indian J. Plant Path,* **7**: 83-84.

Gupta, M.L., Singh, H.B., Kalra, A., Pandey, R. and Singh, S.P. 1997. A new leaf spot of senna caused by *Colletotrichum gloeosporioides. Indian J. Plant Pathol.* **15**: 95-96.

Gupta, S., Kumar, A. and Thakur, R.N. 1993. Some problems in cultivation of *Withania somnifera (L) Dunel (Aswagandha)* in Jammu region of India. *J. Res. Edu. Ind. Med.* **12**: 23-27.

Gutnikova, Z.I. 1963. *Ginseng and its cultivation*, Primorskoe Knizhnoe izd-vo, Vladivostok. 123 pp (Russian).

Halfan-Meir, H. 1973. *Alternaria crassa* a seed-borne fungus of Datura. *Plant Dis. Reptr.* **57:** 960-963.

Hamilton, M.A. 1932. Three new virus diseases of *Hyosycamus niger – Ann. Appl. Biol.* **9**: 550-567.

Hammond, J. 1981. Viruses occurring in *Plantago* species in England. *Plant Pathology* **30**: 237-243.

Handa, S.S. 1992. Medicinal plants based drug industry and emerging plant drugs. CROMAP, **14**: 233-262.

Haseeb, A. and Pandey, R. 1989. Root-knot disease of henbane, *Hyoscyamus* – a new disease record. *Trop. Pest Management,* 35: 212-213.

Haseeb, A., Pandey, R. and Husain, A. 1983. Some new host record of root-knot nematode, *Meloidogyne incognita* (Kofoid & White) Chitwood. *Curr. Sci.* **53**: 1151-52.

Holcomb, G.E. 1998. First report of *Choanephora* flower spot and blight of periwinkle. *Plant Dis* **82**: 447.

Horompoli, T. 1988. Fusarium dry rot *Fusarium oxysporum* Schl. a new disease of poppy (*Papaver somniferum*) in Hungary. *Novenyvedlem* **24**: 201-207.

Horvath, J. and Besada, W.H. 1975. Opium poppy (*Papaver somniferum* L.) – a new natural host of turnip mosaic virus in Hungary. *Z. Pflanzenschvtz.* **82:** 162.

Husain, A. and Janardhanan, K.K. 1967. Effect of seed dressing fungicides on germination of belladonna *Labdev. J. Sci. Technol.* **5:** 158.

Husain, A. *Medicinal plants and their cultivation,* Central Institute of Medicinal and Aromatic Plants, Lucknow, 1993, pp. 111.

Jain, N.K. 1987. Status Report on diseases of Palmarosa and Liquorice. *Proc. AICRP (M&AP) Nov. 2-5, 1987, Udaipur.* p. 367.

Jain, N.K. Status report of diseases in MP. *Proc. V. All India Workshop on MAP,* Bangalore, 22-25 Dec., 1985.

Janardhanan, K.K. and Husain, A. 1967. A new disease of *Lochnera rosea. Labdev J. Sci. Technol* **5**: 69-70.

Janardhanan, K.K. and Husain, A. 1969. Production of hydrolytic and transeliminative enzymes by *Fausarium oxysporium f. sp. rauvolfii. Plant Science* **1**: 136-142.

Janardhanan, K.K. and Husain, A. 1972. A new *Alternaria* blight of *Datura innoxia* Mill. *Indian Phytopath.* **25**: 461-463.

Janardhanan, K.K. and Husain, A. 1974. Production of a toxic metabolite and pectolytic enzyme by *Pythium butleri. Mycopath. Mycol appl.* **52**: 325-330.

Janardhanan, K.K. and Husain, A. 1975. Isolation of tenuazonic acied, a phyhtotoxin from *Alternaria alternata* causing leaf blight of *Datura innoxia* Mill. *Indian J. Exp. Biol.* **13**: 321-322.

Janardhanan, K.K. and Husain, A. 1983. Studies on isolation, purification and identification of tenuazonic acid, a phytotoxin produced by *Alternaria alternata* (Fr) Keissler causing leaf blight of *Datura innoxia* Mill. *Mycopathologia* **83**: 135-140.

Janardhanan, K.K. and Husain, A. 1984. Phytotoxic activity of tenuazonic acid isolated from *Alternaria alternata* (Fr) Keissler causing leaf blight of *Datura innoxia* Mill. and its effect on host metabolism. *Phytopath Z.* **111**: 305-311.

Janardhanan, K.K., Ganguly, D. and Husain, A. 1964. Fusarium wilt of *Rauvolfia serpentina. Curr. Sci.* **33**: 313.

Janardhanan, K.K., Gupta, M.L. and Husain, A. 1977. *Pythium* die-back, a new disease of *Catharanthus roseus* (L.) G. Don., *Indian Phytopath.* **39**: 427-430.

Janardhanan, K.K.; Husain, A. and Khan, M.A. 1971. A new *Pythium root-rot of Belladonna. Plant Sci.* **3**: 119-120.

Jankulowa, M. Huth, W; Wittmann, G. and Paul, H.L. 1968. Untersuchungen uber ein neues isometrisches virus aus *Atropa belladonna* L. II Serologische reaktionen basenverhaltuisse der RNS und aminosaurenzusammen setzung des proteins. *Phytopath. Z.* **63**: 177-185.

Joshi, H.U. and Raychaudhari, S.P. 1964. Mosaic disease of Periwinkle (*Vinca rosea* (L.)). *Indian J. Hort.* **21**: 257-261.

Kalara, A., Ravindra, N.S. and Chandrasekhara, R.S. 1991. Influence of foliar application of fungicides and alkaloid yield of periwinkle (*Catharanthus roseus*) *Indian J. Agri. Sci.* **61**: 949-951.

Kapoor, J.N. and Chowdhary, P.N. 1976. Notes on Indian microfungi. *Indian Phytopath* **29**: 348-352.

Kar, R.K., Kabir, T. and Patnaik, H. 1983. Chemotherapy of periwinkle little leaf disease. *Curr. Sci.* **52**: 486-497.

Kar, R.K., Nanda, H.P. and Kabi, T. 1982. A little leaf of *Catharanthus roseus* in India. *Sci Cult.* **48**: 180-182.

Khadr, A.S. and Abdel-Karer, N.E. 1974. *Alternaria* leaf spot of basil and liquorice, the first report. *Agric. Res. Rev. (Cairo),* **52**: 85-88.

Khan, A.S. and Kamul. M. 1982. Note on *Cercospora cavarae* P&D. Saccardo. *Curr. Sci.* **31**: 341-342.

Khatua, D.C. and Maiti, S. 1982. Two new leaf blight diseases caused by *Rhizoctonia solani. Indian Phytopath.* **35**: 124-25.

Kheswalla, K.F. 1935. Seedling blight of *Cinchona ledgeriana* Moens caused by *Phytophthora palmivora.* Butl. in the Darjeeling district. *Indian. Agr. Sci.* **5**: 455-495.

Khristova, A. 1943. Fungi causing spots on the balls and moulding the seed of opium poppy. *J. Agric. Exp. Stn.* Bulgaria **13**: 13.

Kishoi, K. 1988. *Plant diseases in Japan.* Zenkokeu Nosonkyoiken Kyobai Co. Ltd., Tokyo 943 pp. (Japanese).

Koch, W. 1964. Helminthosporium leaf spot of *Dioscorea* in Guatemala. *Phytopathology* **54**: 365-366.

Kochman, J. 1936. The smut fungi of Poland. *Planta Polon.* **4**: 1.

Koenig, R. 1976. A loop-structure in the serological classification system of tymoviruses. *Virology,* **72**: 1-5.

Kothari, K.L. and Prasad, N. 1970. Downy mildew of opium poppy in Rajasthan. *Indian Phytopath.* **23**: 674-688.

Kothari, K.L. and Prasad, N. 1972. Powdery mildew of opium poppy in Rajasthan and its control. *Indian Phytopath.* **25**: 36.

Kothari, K.L. and Verma, A.C. 1967. Control of downy mildew of opium poppy by root application of fungicides. *Pl. Dis. Rep* **51**: 686.

Kotin, Yu. A. and Protsenko, A.E. 1973. Mosaic virus of *Datura metel* L. *Byulleten Glavnogo Botanicheskogo Sada.* **87**: 113-115.

Kovachevaky, J.C. and Kovachevsky, I.C. 1968. Bean yellow mosaic virus in Bulgaria. *Phytopath. Z.* **61**:41.

Kovachevski, I. 1974. Virus wilt of thorn apple in Bulgaria. *Rasteniev dni Nauki* **11**: 128-136.

Kovachevsky, I.C. 1936. Parasitic fungi new for Bulgaria, Fourth Contribution. *Tran. Soc. Bulg. Sci. Nat* **17**: 13.

Kowalski , J. 1968. Investigations on some biological properties of fungi attacking leaves of *Digitalis purpurea* and *D. lanata. Acta mycol. Warszawa* **4:** 25-38.

Kulkarni, R.N. and Ravindra, N.S. 1988. Resistance fo *Pythium aphanidermatum* diploid and induced tetraploids of *Catharanthus roseus. Planta Medica* **54**: 356-359.

Kulkarni, R.N. and Ravindra, N.S. 1997. Integration of host resistance with fungicide in the control of die-back disease of periwinkle. *Tropical Agriculture* **74**: 321-323.

Kulkarni, R.N., Kalra, A. and Ravindra, N.S. 1992. Integration of soil solarization with host resistance in the control of die-back and collar and root rot disease of periwinkle. *Tropical Agri.* **69**: 217-222.

Kumar, S. Shukla, R.S. Singh, K.P.a nd Husain, A. 1982. Leaf blight of *Hyoscyamus niger* in India. *Indian Phytopath.* **35**: 335.

Kumar, S., Shukla, R.S., Singh, K.P. and Husain, A. 1984. *Alternaria* leaf spot disease of *Hyoscyamus muticus* in India. *Indian J. Mycol. Pl. Path.* **14**: 176.

Kumawat, H. 1979. Grow isabgul as a commercial crop. *Farmer and Parliament* **10**: 21-23.

Legha. P.K., Sharma, G.D. and Gupta, R., Liquorice. *In: Advances in Horticulture. Vol. 11. Medicinal and Aromatic Plants.* K.L. Chadha and R. Gupta (Ed.), Malhotra Publishing House, New Delhi, 1995.

Latysheva. T.A. and Sevriuk. N.I. 1981. *Ginseng diseases.* Zashchita rastenii 'Kolos' **11**: 23-24 (Russian).

Lee, R.F., Niblett, C.L.; Hubhard, J.D. and Johnson, L.B. 1979. Characterization of belladonna mottle virus isolates from Kansas and Iowa. *Phytopathology,* **69**: 985-989.

Lele, C.V. and Ashram. 1968. Die-back disease of *Rauvolfia serpentina* Benth caused by *Colletotrichum dematium. Indian Phytopath.* **20**: 349-350.

Letieritz, R. and Rodder, W. 1980. On important plant protection methods in expanded cultivation of opium poppy in the Dresden district. *Nachrichtenblatt. Pflanzenschutz.* DDR **34**: 166.

Li. H.K. and Yang. C.H. 1988. *Cultivation and processing of gi 1seng.* Fashing Chi-lin sheng hsinhua Shin tien, Beijing 239 pp (Chinese).

Mahrishi, R.P. 1986. *Withania somnifera* a new host of *Myrothecium roridum. Ind. J. Mycol. Pl. Pathol.* **16**: 199.

Maiti, S. and Chattopadhyay, S.B. 1986. Studies on diseases of Indian medicinal plants – II. *Indian J. Mycol. Res.* **24**: 103-111.

Masalab, N.A. 1938. Diseases of medicinal and some industrial plants caused by *Sclerotinia. Sovitsk. Bot*: 67-83.

Masurat, G and Stephan, S. 1961. The occurrence of the most important diseases and pests of crop and garden plants in 1960 in German Democratic Republic. *Nachr. Bl. dtsch. Pfl. Sch Dienst. Berl. NF.* **15**: 125.

Matuo, T. and Miyazawa. Y. 1984. Scientific name of *Cylindrocrpon* sp causing root rot of ginseng. *Annls. Phytopath Soc.* (Japan). **50**: 649-652.

McClean, A.P.D. and Cowin, S.M. 1952. Diseases of crucifers and other plants caused by cabbage ring spot virus. *Sci. Bull. Dep. Agric. S. Afri.* **332**: 30.

McGovern, R.J. 1994. Target spot of *Catharanthus roseus* caused by *Corynespora casiicola*. *Plant Dis.* **78**: 83.

McPartland, J. and Hosoya, T. 1998. Species of *Colletotrichum* on ginseng (*Panax*) *Mycotaxon* **67**: 3-8.

McPartland, J.M. 1985. Organisms isolated from soil previously planted in American ginseng. Fromm Brothers, Inc. (Hamburg. WI) *Technical Report, Supplement,* 5 pp.

McRae, W. 1930. Report of Imperial Mycologist. *Sci. Rep. Agric. Res . Inst. Pusa*, 1928-29. pp. 51-66.

McRae, W. 1933. *Report of Agric. Res. Inst. Pusa.* 1931-32, pp. 122-140.

McRae. W. 1932. *Report of Agric. Res. Inst. Pusa.* 1930-31. pp. 73-86.

Meffert, M.E. 1949. On the history of the helminthosporiosis of the opium poppy. *Nachr. Bl. dtsch. Pfl. Sch. Dienst. Berl. N.F.* **3**: 104.

Mehrotra, M.D. 1976. Studies on some interesting diseases of *Rauvolfia serpentina* form India. I. Contribution to the knowledge of disease development on relation to environment. *Indian Forester*. **102**: 119-125.

Mehrotra, M.D. and Thapar, H.S. 1990. *Rhizoctonia* leaf spotting and blight of *Rauvolfia serpentina* a new disease from India. *Indian Forester*. **116**: 372-374.

Mehta, N., Madan, R.L. and Thakur, D.P. 1985. Record of isabgol wilt from Haryana. *Haryana Agric. Univ. J.* **15**: 473-474.

Miczulska, I. 1967. Observation on the influence of infection of poppy (*P. somniferum* L.) by parasitic fungi on the morphine content in the poppy heads. *Roczn. Nauk. Roln. Ser. A. Rosl.* **93:** 189.

Middleton, J.T. 1943. *Phytophthora* rot of belladonna. *Bull. Torrey. Bot. Club* **70**: 244-257.

Miltovic, I. 1952. Contribution to the knowledge of the fungus *Pleospora clavescens* (Fr.) Tulasne on poppy. *Rev. Sci. Agric. Zogreb.* **13**: 121.

Miller, P.R., Weiss. F. and O. Brien. M.J. 1960. *Index of plant diseases in the United States.* Agricultural Handbook No.165 U.S.D.A., Washington, D.C. 531 pp.

Minz, G. and Harari, D.S. 1969. Additional host plants of root-knot nematode, *Meloidogyne* Spp recorded in Israel during 1963-1968. *Isr. J. Agric Res.* **19**: 137-138.

Misko, L.A. 1963. Helminthosporiosis of poppy *Zashch Rasi Moskva* **8:** 56.

Moesz, G. 1938. Fungi of Hungary II: Archimycetes and Phycomycetes. *Ann. Hist. nat. Mus. Hung.* **31:** 109.

Mohanthy, N.N. and Addy, S.K. 1957. *Cercospora* leaf spot of *Rauvolfia serpentina* Benth. *Curr. Sci.* **26**: 289-290.

Mohanty, N.N. and Addy, S.K. 1958. Target spot of *Rauvolfia serpentina. Sci.. Cult..* **23**: 608-609.

Moline H.E. and Fries, R.E., 1974. A strain of belladonna mottle virus isolated from *Physalis hetrophylla* in Iowa. *Phytopathology* **64**: 44-48.

Mraz, F. 1960. The influence of the harmful effect of the fungus *Helminthosporium papaveris* on poppy yields in the regions Karlovy-vary in the years 1957 and 1958. *Ann. Acad. Tichecosl Agric* **93:** 1083.

Mraz, F. 1963. Study of the effectiveness of treatment compound on the conidia of the fungus *Helminthosporium papaveris* (Henning). *Ann. Acad. Tchecost. Agric.* **36:** 51.

Muller, H.M. Sorguceva, N.A. Fedotina, V.L. Schmidt, H.B. Kleinhempel, H. Procenko, A.E. and Spaar, D. 1974. Investigations in the USSR and GDR on the electron microscopic detection of mycoplasma like organisms in plants. *Archiv. Fur. Phytopathologic und Pflanznschutz.* **10:** 15.

Nagaraja, S. Kulkarni, S., Hegde, R.K. and Kulkarni, S. 1992. Physiological studies on *Drechslera sorokiniana* (Sacc) Subram & Jain, a causal agent of leaf spot of *Dioscorea* Sp. *Mysore J. Agric. Sci.* **26**: 261-264.

Nagaraja, S., Kulkarni, S. and Hegde, R.K. 1980. A new leaf spot of *Dioscorea composita* in India. *Ind. Phytopath.* **33**: 518-519.

Nair V.M.G. 1991. Recent advances in ginseng (*Panax* spp) research and the importance of germplasm of wild medicinal plants. In *Recent Advances in Medicinal, Aromatic & Spices Crops* Vol 1 (Ed. S.P. Raychaudhuri) Today & Tomorrow's Printers and Publishers, New Delhi, 39-51.

Nakata, K. and Takimoto, S. 1922. Studies on ginseng diseases in Korea. *Bull. Agric. Exper. Sta. Govern. Gen Shosen* (Korea) **5**: 1-17 (Japanese).

Narain, U. 1990. New record of *Alternaria papaveris* from India. *Indian Phytopath.* **43:** 147.

Navarro de Palencia, J. 1954. The attacks of *Fusarium* on the opium poppy. *Bot. Inst. Invest. agron. Madr.* **14:** 377-381.

Nienhaus. F. 1960. Das wirthsspektru n von *Phytophthora cactorum* (Leb. et Cohn) Sehroter. *Phytopathol. Z.* **38**: 33-68.

Nigam, K.B. 1984. Asgandh cultivation. *Indian Horticulture,* Special issue, pp. 39-41.

Nikitina, K.V. and Kauhrusheva, T.E. 1975. Fungal and bacterial diseases of opium poppy in the Leningrad district. *Trudy Prik. Bot. Gen. Selekt.* **55:** 224-229.

Ohh, S.H. 1981. Diseases of ginseng: Environmental and host effect on disease out break and growth of pathogens. *Korean J. Ginseng Sci.* **5**: 73-84.

Padwick. G.W. and Merch, J.L. 1943. Notes on Indian Fungi I *Mycological paper* No.7, CMI, Kew, U.K.

Pandey, G.N. 1987. Chemical control of *Withania somnifera. Biannual Workshop,* Udaipur.

Pandey, G.N. 1988. Symptomatology and control of Asgandh diseases. *Nat. Sem. Med. Arom. Pl.* Indore.

Pandey, G.N. 1995. Diseases management of medicinal plants. In: *Advances in Horticulture* Vol.II. *Medicinal and Aromatic Plants* K.L. Chadha and Rajendra Gupta (Eds.) Malhotra Publishing House, New Delhi, India. pp. 249-269.

Pandey, G.N. and Nigam, K.B. 1985. *Annual Workshop, All India Co-ordinated project on medicinal and aromatic plants,* Bangalore-22-25 Dec.

Pandey, G.N. and Nigam, K.B. 1986. Studies on symptomatology and control of downy mildew in opium poppy. *Symp. Agric. Develop. Nimar* and *Malwa.* Indore.

Pandey, G.N. Disease management of Medicinal Plants. In: *Advances in Horticulture Vol 11 Medicinal and Aromatic Plants.* K.L. Chadha and R. Gupta, Melhotra Publishing House, New Delhi, 1995. p. 249-269.

Pandey, G.N., Nigam, K.B. and Kandalkar, V.I. 1985. A new record of die-back of Asgandha (*Withania somnifera* Durel) *Tec. Session. V. All India Workshop on M&AP,* Bangalore, 22-25.

Pandotra, V.R. and Husain, A. 1966. Fungi on medicinal and aromatic plants in the north west Himalayas.IV. *Mycopath. Mycol. appl.* **29**: 155-159.

Pareek, S.K., Srivastava, V.K., Maheshwari, M.L., Singh, S. and Gupta, R. 1980. Grow Senna in Northern India. *Indian Farming* **30**: 41-43.

Parisi Rosa. 1921. Notes on some parasites of medicinal and aromatic plants. *Bull. Orto. Bot. Napoli* **6**: 285.

Parke, J.L. and Shortwell. K.M. 1989. Diseases of cultivated ginseng. *Univ. Wis. Madison. Coll. Agric. Life. Sci. Res. Bull.* 3465, 16 pp.

Parker, MA. 1988. Genetic uniformity and disease resistance in a colonal plant. *Amer. Natur.* **132**: 538-549.

Patel, C.C., Patel, H.R., Patel, D.J. and Thakar, N.A. 1989. Relative susceptibility of certain medicinal and aromatic plants to root-knot nematodes. *Pak. J. Nematol* **7**: 81-82.

Patel, D.H., Patel, M.A. and Dalal, K.C. 1991. Effect of length of cutting on root and shoot growth of *Glycyrrhiza. IX-Workshop, AICRP (M&AP), Anand*, P: 296.

Patel, D.J. and Patel, S.J. 1984. Senna an additional host of *Macrophomina plaseolina* in Gujarat. *Indian J. Mycol Plant Pathol* **14**: 293.

Patel, J.C. 1984. Downy mildew of isabgul (*Plantago ovata* Forsk). *Doctoral Thesis, Gujarat Agricultural Univ. Anand*, India.

Patel, J.C. and Desai, M.V. 1987. New disease outbreak (leaf blight of *Plantago ovata*). *Indian Phytopath.* **37**: 582.

Patel, K.D. and Pillai, S.N. 1979. Effect of leaf spot disease on sennoside content in senna leaves. *Indian Drugs* **17**: 1-2.

Paul, H.L., Bode, O., Jankulowa, M. and Brandes, J. 1968. Untersuchungen uber ein neues isometrisches virus aus *Atropa belladonna* L. I Symptomatologie reingung, morphologie, physikausche und chemische eigenschaftein. *Phytopath. Z.* **61**: 342-361.

Paul, Y.S. and Bhardwaj, L.N. 1992. Phyllosticta leaf spot of *Glycyrrhiza glabra* Linn. A new disease from India. *Indian Forester.* **118**: 301-302.

Pavgi, M.S. and Upadhyay. 1964. Parasitic fungi from North India, II. *Mycopasth Mycol. appl.* **24**: 347.

Pelikanova, J., Petrizik, K. and Honestslegrova, J. 1992. The discovery of belladonna mottle virus in Czechoslovakia and its comparison with Hungarian isolate of this virus. *J. Phytopathology*, **134**: 10-16.

Phatak, H.C. and Raychoudhary, S.P. 1967. *Withania somnifera* – additional host of tobacco leaf curl virus. *Sci. Cult.* **33**: 234-235.

Phillips, S., Piggott, J.D.A. and Brunt, A.A. 1986. Further evidence that *Dioscorea* latent virus is a potex virus. *Ann. Appl. Biol.* **109**: 137-145.

Piccirillo, P. and Caponigro, V. 1992. A tobacco isolate of tobacco mosaic virus (TMV), systemic on *Datura metel*. *Petria* **2**: 11-17.

Pillai, S.N. and Patel, K.D. 1982. Leaf spot of Senna – A new record. *Indian J. Mycol Plant Pathol* **12**: 54.

Polezinski, L. 1982. Ginseng (*Panax quinquefolius* L) culture in Marathon Country, Wisconsin, *M.S. thesis, University of Wiscongin* at Stevens Point, 143 pp.

Porth, A., Lessmann, D.E. and Vetten, H.J. 1987. Characterization of Poty-virus isolates from West Africans Yam (*Dioscorea* Spp.) *J. Phytopathology*, **120**: 166-183.

Prasanna, G.B., Rajeswari, A., Satyanarayanan, T., Kiranmai, G., Gopinath, K., Sreenivas, P. and Nayudu, M.V. 1996. Characterization of virus causing leaf distortion disease of *Datura metel* in India. *Indian J. Virology* **12**: 129-135.

Prochaska, M. 1928. Observations on the occurrence of *Peronospora arborescens* (downy mildew) on *Papaver somniferum. Fortschr. der Landw.* 3: 165.

Proctor, C.H. 1944. A virus disease of henbane (*Hyoscyamus niger*) in New Zealand. *N.Z. J. Sci. Tech* – A **26**: 83-87.

Proctor, J.T.A, Lee, J.C. and Lee, S.S. 1990. Ginseng production in Korea. *Hort. Sci.* **25**: 746-754.

Radulescu, E. and Perseca. E. 1964. On the biology of *P. papaveraceae. Rev. Roum. Biol. Ser. Bot.* **9:** 19.

Radulescu, E. Perseca. E. and Docea, E. 1961. Contribution to the control of helminthosporiosis of poppies (*P. clavescens)* by agrotechnical and chemical methods. *Lucr. Stiit. Inst. Agron. N. Balescu Ser B* : **5: 333.**

Rajendran, G. and Vadivelu, S. 1991. Pathogenicity of *Meloidogyne incognita* to *Coleus forskohlii. J. Root Crops* **17**: 210-211.

Ramakrishnan, T.S. 1949. The occurrence of *Pythium vexans* de Bary in South India. *Indian Phytopath.* **2**: 27-30.

Ramakrishnan, T.S. 1951. Addition to fungi of Madras X. *Proc. Indian Acad. Sci. B.* **34**: 63-72.

Ravindra, N.S. 1988. Root and collar rot of *Catharanthus roseus* caused by *Pythium aphanidermatum*. *Indian. J. Mycol Plant Path.* **16**: 288.

Reddy, M.A.R., Tewari, R.K. and Bakshi, B.K. 1971. Target leaf-spot disease of *Rauvolfia serpentina* and its chemical control. *Indian For.* **97**: 487-492.

Reed. H.R. 1905. Three fungus diseases of the cultivated ginseng. *Missouri Agric. Exp. Stat. Bull.* No. **69**, pp. 45-66.

Reinmuth, E. 1942. Parasitic leaf desiccation, a noteworthy disease in poppy cultivation. *Angew Bot.* **24:** 273.

Rudny, R. 1976. The effect of sowing time, methods of cultivation and protective measures on the health and yield of opium poppy (*Papaver somniferum* L.) variety Mak niebieski K.M. *Prace Naukowe Instytutu Ochrony Roslin* 18: 167.

Russell, T.F. 1975. *Plantago wilt. Phytopathology,* **65**: 359-360.

Saini, S., Sattar, A. and Alam, M. 1996. Occurrence of stem-rot disease caused by *Rhizopus stolonifer* on periwinkle. *Indian. J. Plant Pathol.* **14**: 1-4.

Sastry, K.S.M. 1972. Mosaic virus complex of *Digitalis lanata* Ehrh. *Ind. J. Microbiol,* **11**: 125-126.

Sastry, K.S.M. 1973. Studies on virus disease of some medicinal plants. *Indian J. Hort.* **30**: 562-566.

Sastry, K.S.M., Thakur, R.N. and Pandotra, V.R. Diseases of medicinal and aromatic plants and their control. In: *Cultivation and utilization of medicinal and aromatic plants.* Regional Research Laboratory, Jammu-Tawi, 1977, 711-733.

Sattar, A. Janardhanan, K.K. and Husain, A. 1988. Bacteriual stem rot of opium poppy caused by *Erwinia carotovora* sub sp. *carotovora. FAO Plant Prot. Bull* **36**: 163-164.

Sattar, A., Alam, M. and Janardhanan, K.K. 1986. Isolation of tenuazonic acid, a phytotoxin from *Alternaria crassa* (Sacc) Rands causing leaf blight and fruit rot of *Datura stramonium* Mill. *Curr. Sci.* **55**: 195-196.

Sattar, A., Janardhanan, K.K. and Husain, A. 1986. Bacterial blight of Egyptian henbane. *FAO Plant Prot. Bull* – **34:** 161.

Sattar, A., Singh, H.B., Saini, S. and Alam, M. 1995. Occurrence of *Sclerotinia sclerotiorum* on important medicinal and aromatic plants. *Indian. J. Plant Pathol* **13**: 1-5.

Savulescu, T. 1932. Phytosanitary conditions in Romania during the year 1930-31. *Inst. Cerc. Agron. al Romaniei Publ.* **8**: 31.

Sawada, K. 1936. Phytophthora blight of cinchona seedlings occurring in Formosa caused by *Phytophthora cinchonae* Saw n. sp. *Formosan Agr. Rev* **32**: 316-346.

Schumann, K. 1963. Untersuchnugen zur charakterisierung und identifizierung der erreger des Digitalis mosaic 1. Das tabakmosaikvirus (*Marmor tabaci* H). *Phytopath Z.* **48**: 1-28.

Sehgal, S.P., Gupta, P.J. and Agarwala, J.M. 1971. Capsule rot of opium poppy (*Papaver somniferum* L.) *Rajasthan J. Agric. Sci.* **2**: 61.

Shakhela, R.R., Jose V.T. and Tikka, S.B.S. 1985. It is paying to grow isabgul. *Farmers and Parliament* **20**: 22, 32.

Sharma, A.D.and Jandiak, C.L. 1979. *Rhizoctonia* disease of *Atropa* and *Salvia* new to India. *Indian J. Mycol. Plant Pathol.* **9**: 86-87.

Sharma, A.K., Misra, S., Kumar, K. and Cousin, T. 1993. Association of mycoplasma like organism (MLOs) with naturally infected yellows-diseased periwinkle in India. *International J. Trop. Plant. Dis.* **11**: 91-97.

Shepardson, S. and Mc Green, R.C. 1979. Effect of GA on mycoplasma like organism infected and heatlhy periwinkle. *Plant. Dis. Reptr.* **63**: 965-869.

Shin, H.S. Lee. H.H. and Lee. M.W. 1986. Studies on the distribution of fungal and *Fusarium* spp. Propagules in ginseng field soil. *Korean J. Mycol.* **14**: 109-119.

Shoemaker, P.B. and Konsler, T.R. 1982. Fungicide evaluation for *Alternaria* blight of ginseng 1981. Fungal nematicide tests. *Am. Phytopath Soc.* **73**: 54.

Sholberg. P.L., Li.T. and Ginns. J. 1996. First report of powdery mildew on ginseng in North America. *Plant Dis.* **80**: 463.

Shukla, R.S., Kumar, S., Singh, H.N. and Singh, K.P. 1993. First report of aerial blight of *Coleus forskohlii* caused by *Rhizoctonia solani* in India. *Plant. Dis.* **77**: 429.

Shukla, R.S., Kumar, S., Singh, K.P. and Husain, A. 1988. Seedling blight of *Hyoscyamus muticus* by *Pythium butleri* in India. *Curr. Sci.* **57**: 40.

Singh, G. and Singh, R.N. 1984. Leaf spot disease of *Atropa belladonna. Indian Phytopath,* **37**: 585.

Singh, G., Singh, R.N. and Bisht, I.S. 1985. Control of leaf spot disease of belladonna caused by *Ascochyta atropae*. *Indian Phytopath*, **38**: 183-184.

Singh, H.B., Gupta, M.L., Pandey, R., Kalra, A. and Singh, S.P. 1996. A new leaf blight of Senna caused by *Alternaria cassiae*. *Indian J. Plant Path.* **14**: 71-72.

Singh, S. 1980. Datura leaf distortion mosaic of cucumber mosaic virus. *Indian Phytopath.* **34**: 92-94.

Sivakumar, C.V. and Vidhyasekaran, P. 1990. Control of *Meloidogyne incognita* on *Coleus forskohlii* with *Paeciliomyces bilacinus* in farm yard manure amended and non-amended soil *J. Biol Control* **4**: 68-69.

Smith, K.M. 1943. A virus disease of *Atropa belladonna*. *Parasitology*, **35**: 1590-160.

Smith, K.M. 1945. A further note on the viruses affecting *Atropa belladonna* and a description of virus complex affecting *Hyoscyamus niger*. *Parasitology*, **36**: 209-210.

Sohn, J.J. and Plicansky, D. 1977. The costs of reproduction in the mayapple *Podophyllum peltatum* (Berberidaceae) *Ecology* **58**: 1366-1374.

Sol, H.H. Van Heuven, J.C. and Seinhorst, J.W. 1961. Transmission of rattle virus and *A. belladonna* mosaic virus by nematodes. *Tijdschr. Plantziekten.* **66**: 228-231.

Spak, J. and Kubelkova, D. 1990. Occurrence of turnip mosaic virus in opium (*Papaver somniferum* L.) in Czechoslovakia. *Sbornik UVTI Z.* **26**: 257-261.

Stefanac, Z., Gailhofer, M., Thaler, I and Mamula, D. 1993. Some characteristics of crystalline inclusions associated with henbane mosaic potyvirus. *Acta Botanica Croatica.* **52**: 1-4.

Subba-Rao, B.L., Husain, A. and Manohar, S.K. 1983. Association of mycoplasma like bodies in little leaf disease of periwinkle (*Catharanthus roseus*) in India. *Indian. J. Plant. Pathol.* **1**: 122-124.

Subba-Rao, B.L. and Husain, A. 1984. Green mosaic : A virus disease of *Hyoscyamus muticus* L. in India. *Curr. Sci.* **53**: 482-483.

Sundraraman, S. 1928. Administrative report of the government Mycologist Coimbatore. *Rep. Dept. Agric. Madras*, 1927-28, pp. 355-372.

Szkolnik, M. 1951. *Phytophthora parasitica* disease of cinchona in Central American field planting. *Pl. Dis. Reptr.* **35**: 16-24.

Takimoto, S. 1919. *Colletotrichum panacicola* Uyeda & Takimoto. *Chozen Nokwai ho* **14**: 24-25 (in Japanese).

Thakore, B.B.L., Jain, J.P., Singh, R.B., Khandelwal, G.L. and Mathur, S. 1983. Loss due to downy mildew of opium poppy and its reduction by application of fungicides. *Indian Phytopath* **36**: 442-44.

Thakur, R.N. 1974. Root and foot-rot of *Datura innoxia* caused by *Corticium solani* . *Indian Phytopath* **27**: 129-130.

Thakur, R.N. and Sastry, K.S.M. 1970. Studies on *Sclerotium* root-rot of *Datura innoxia* Mill. *Labdev. J. Sci. Technol* 8 B: 115-116.

Thakur, R.N. and Bhat, B.K. 1980. *Phytophthora* root-rot of *Atropa belladonna* in Kashmir Valley. *Indian J. Mycol. Plant Path.* **9**: 82.

Thomas, C.A. 1951. Anthracnose of Digitalis. *Phytopathology* **41**: 997-1000.

Thomas, J.E. and Dietzgen. R.G. 1991. Characterization of Datura yellow vein virus, a newly described rhabdo virus from Australia. *Annal. Appl. Biol.* **118**: 339-349.

Thompson, A. 1939. Notes on plant disease in 1939. *Malayan. Agr. Jour.* **28**: 400-407.

Tomlinson, J.A. Webb, M.J.W. and Elizabeth, M.F. 1972. Studies on broccoli necrotic yellow virus. *Ann. Appl. Biol.* **71**: 127-34.

Turkoglu, T. 1979. Mosaic virus of opium poppy in Turkey. *J. Turk. Phytopath.* **8**: 77.

Turkuede, B.B., Singh, R. Lambat, A.K. and Khule, W.B. 1982. Fungicidal control of downy mildew of opium poppy. *Pesticides* **16**: 21-22.

Varadarajan, P.D. 1958. Blight and die-back disease of *Rauvolfia serpentia. J. Biol.* **1: 1-4**.

Varadarajan, P.D. 1964. Anthracnose disease of *Rauvolfia serpentina* Benth. caused by *Colletotrichum gleosporioides* Perz. *Curr. Sc.* **33**: 564-565.

Varadarajan, P.D. 1966. Leaf spot and premature defoliation of *Raufolfia serpentina* Benth. under cultivation caused by *Curvularia lunata* (Wakker) Boed. *Indian Phytopathol* **19**: 298-300.

Varadarajan, P.D. 1967. Bunchy top 'virus' of *Rauvolfia serpentina*. *Indian Phytopath.* **20**: 255-257.

Verma, H.N. and Dwivedi, K. 1991. A distortion mosaic disease of *Catharanthus roseus*. *Recent. Adv. Med. Arom. Spice Crops*, 155-158.

Walkey, D.G.A., Spence, N.J. Clay, C.M. and Miller A. 1994. A potyvirus isolated from solanaceous hosts. *Plant Pathology* **43**: 431-437.

Whetzel, H.H. , Jackson, H.S. and Mains, E.B. 1925. The composite life history of *Puccinia podophylli* Schw *J. Agric. Res.* **30**: 65-79.

Winters, H.F. 1950. Prevention of damping-off in cinchona seedling beds. *Trop. Agric.* **27:** 123-126.

Winters, H.F. 1951. Fumigation of Cinchona nursery soil. *Turrialba Rev. Inst. Cionc. Agric.* **1**: 296-298.

Yaraguntaiah, R.C. and Govindu, H.C. 1972. Studies on a mosaic disease of *Datura metel* Linn. in Mysore. *Mysore J. Agric. Sci.* **6**: 352-356.

Yossifovitch, M. 1928. Kingdom of the Serbs, Croates and Solvenes: A destructive disease of the poppy in Southern Serbia. *Internat. Bull. Plant Protect.* **11**: 18.

Yossifovitch, M. 1929. *Peronospora arborescens* (Berk) de Bary, a very important parasite of *Papaver somniferum* in Yugoslavia. *Rev. Path. Veg. et Int. Agric* **16**: 235.

Zaidi, A.A., Singh, B.P. and Srivastava, K.M. 1978. Chlorotic stunt, A new virus disease of *Catharanthus roseus* in India. *Curr. Sci.* **47**: 927-928.

Zaim, M and Samad, A. 1995. Association of phytoplasma with witches-broom disease of *Withania somnifera* (L) Durel in India. *Plant Science* **109**: 225-229.

Zaim, M. 1989. A new severe mosaic disease of opium poppy. *Curr. Sci.* **58**: 1095-1096.

Zaim, M. and Khan, M.M.A.A. 1988. Green mosaic of *Hyoscyamus niger* L. and *Rauvolfia serpentina* Benth. ex Kurz. *Indian J. Plant. Pathol.* **6**: 152-157.

Zaman, K.B. and Khan, A.S. 1969. Studies on some disease of *Papaver somniferum* Linn. *Pakistan. J. For.* **19**: 185.

Subject Index

U

V

W

X

Y

Z

AUTHOR INDEX

F

G

H

I

J

K

L

Fig. 64 : Symptoms of witch's broom or phyllody of B. monnieri caused by Phytoplasma (Courtesy of Dr. M. Zaim, CIMAP, Lucknow)

grafting. Treatment of infected plants with tetracycline gave temporary recovery from typical symptoms of the disease after 15-20 days of treatment (Zaim and Samad, 1995).

Causal organism : Phytoplasma (mycoplasma-like organism). Pleomorphic bodies present in the sieve tubes of phloem. The bodies are generally oval, spherical, variable in size ranging between [illegible] nm. They were densely stained and of high electron-opacity and bound by unit membrane. Occasionally found in budding. The organism is highly sensitive to tetracyclines.

Control : Spray with tetracyclines has been recommended for the control of the disease. The recovery of the disease symptoms is often temporary.